It's an
INSIDE JOB

It's an INSIDE JOB

THE FRIEND'S GUIDE TO THE 7 DIMENSIONS OF WELLNESS

Tracy Arnold, Helen Barnard, Diane Hubbard

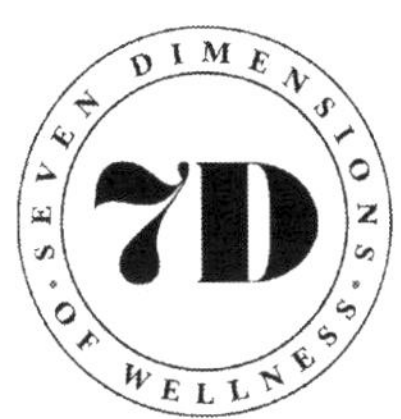

www.sevendimensions.org

Published in the United States by Seven Dimensions of Wellness, LLC, First Printing, 2024

Formatted using Atticus – An Author's Best Friend

ISBN: 979-8-9883899-3-4 (Trade Paper)

ISBN: 979-8-9883899-1-0 (E-Book)

www.sevendimensions.org

This book is dedicated to You, the reader.

You matter.

When you begin to notice the world inside you,

extraordinary things happen.

Foreword

Welcome to a delightful exploration of the different realms of well-being. In the pages that follow, you will embark on an enlightening journey toward a more holistic and joy-filled existence through the seven dimensions. Whether you're a seasoned wellness expert or a curious newcomer, there's something waiting for you within these pages. I invite you to find a cozy spot and join me on a journey of well-being that celebrates the harmonious symphony of mind, body, and soul.

Speaking of symphonies, music has always been a part of my life. I enjoy singing with my family in both formal and informal settings, going to musicals and concerts, or really anywhere that offers a beat, a melody, and most importantly, harmony. Life is a lot like music. It requires rhythm, balance, and sometimes a touch of playfulness to create a beautiful composition. Just as different instruments come together to create a symphony, different aspects of our lives need harmony and balance for us to experience true well-being. Whether it's finding the right intervals between work and play, nourishing our bodies with nutritious food, or cultivating meaningful relationships, every element plays a crucial role in creating a harmonious and fulfilling life.

I'm honored to include a little piece of my story in the pages of this book. The music stopped for me when a devastating wildfire swept through our community and destroyed our home, as well as over a thousand other homes in our town. The flames may have consumed our houses, but they didn't extinguish the essence that binds us. Like a Phoenix rising from the ashes, the spirit of our shared humanity emerged, proving that it is indeed an inside job. I can share with experience that it is in these moments of crisis that we discover our true bravery, resilience, newfound strength, and determination. Despite the challenges we face, we have the power to cultivate resilience, compassion, and growth within ourselves. As a result, music is finding its way back into my life–one beat at a time.

Consider this book a roadmap, or better yet, a treasure map to your own personal well-being, complete with informative signposts, unexpected detours, relatable anecdotes, and practical exercises. Like a compass, it will guide you toward unlocking your inner potential and navigating the ups and downs of life. To me, it feels like a metronome that helps keep me grounded and in rhythm with my own journey. As I turn each page, I am reminded that, just like music, life is a beautiful symphony waiting to be composed. *It's an Inside Job* is a compelling journey that will help you uncover the hidden treasures within yourself, leading you to a path of self-discovery and personal growth.

Here's to embracing the art of living holistically—one grateful heartbeat at a time. Let your rhythm guide you. Happy wandering!
Onward,

Leigh Pierini
Leigh is a PSIA-AASI-RM Examiner, mentor, author, and motivational speaker, always advocating for women's empowerment.

Fun Fact: The repetitive, soothing sound of a metronome can have a calming effect on individuals experiencing anxiety or stress. Listening to the steady rhythm of a metronome can promote relaxation, reduce heart rate, and alleviate tension.

I am your mindset.

I am your well-being.

I am what gives meaning to your life.

I am your relationships.

I am your purpose.

I am the ecosystem in and around you.

I am your guide.

I am you.

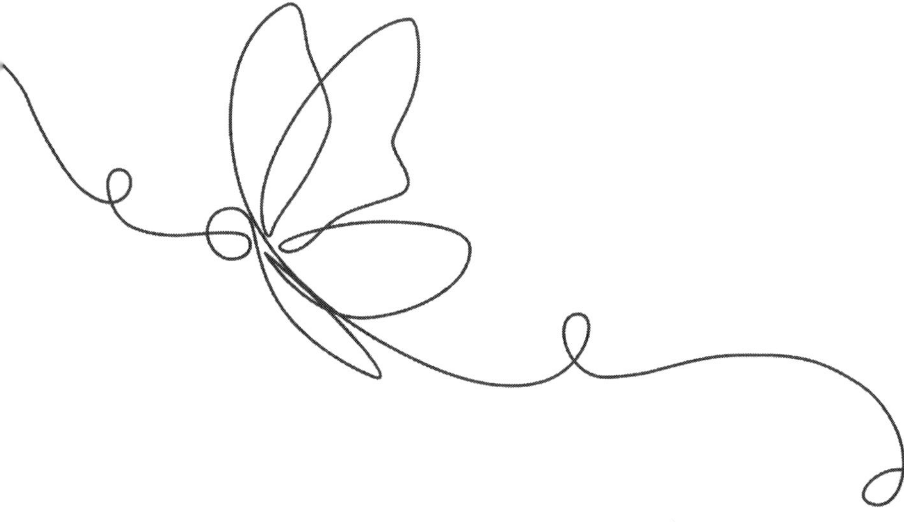

Dear Friend,

This is an invitation to live a healthy, meaningful, and joyful life. What we know for certain is that being well is an inside job; the answers are within us and profoundly unique to each of us. Our body can be the most powerful guide when we learn to tune into its messages. It's time to get out of our minds and into our bodies!

We are excited to have you join our conversation around cultivating a curiosity about ourselves while consciously experiencing life through our seven different yet interconnected dimensions.

When we share our journeys in a safe and supportive environment, our collective knowledge and wisdom help us reach a deeper level of clarity. Living from a place of expanded awareness enables us to make informed choices to create the life we desire. Despite sometimes feeling stuck, discovering that we are all creators of our lives can help us move forward. With self-awareness and self-knowledge, we can access a deep power to heal ourselves.

We understand some of our explorations may not resonate with you; we are sharing from the perspective of our own journeys. Still, we hope you will allow the shared scientific knowledge and personal experiences to spark curiosity and help you take steps toward understanding yourself and what areas of your life need compassion and nourishment.

So come along on a journey to explore what makes us whole. All you need to join us is an open mind and a willingness to feel. Then, it's up to you to take what you need.

Sending you much love,
Tracy, Helen & Diane

Contents

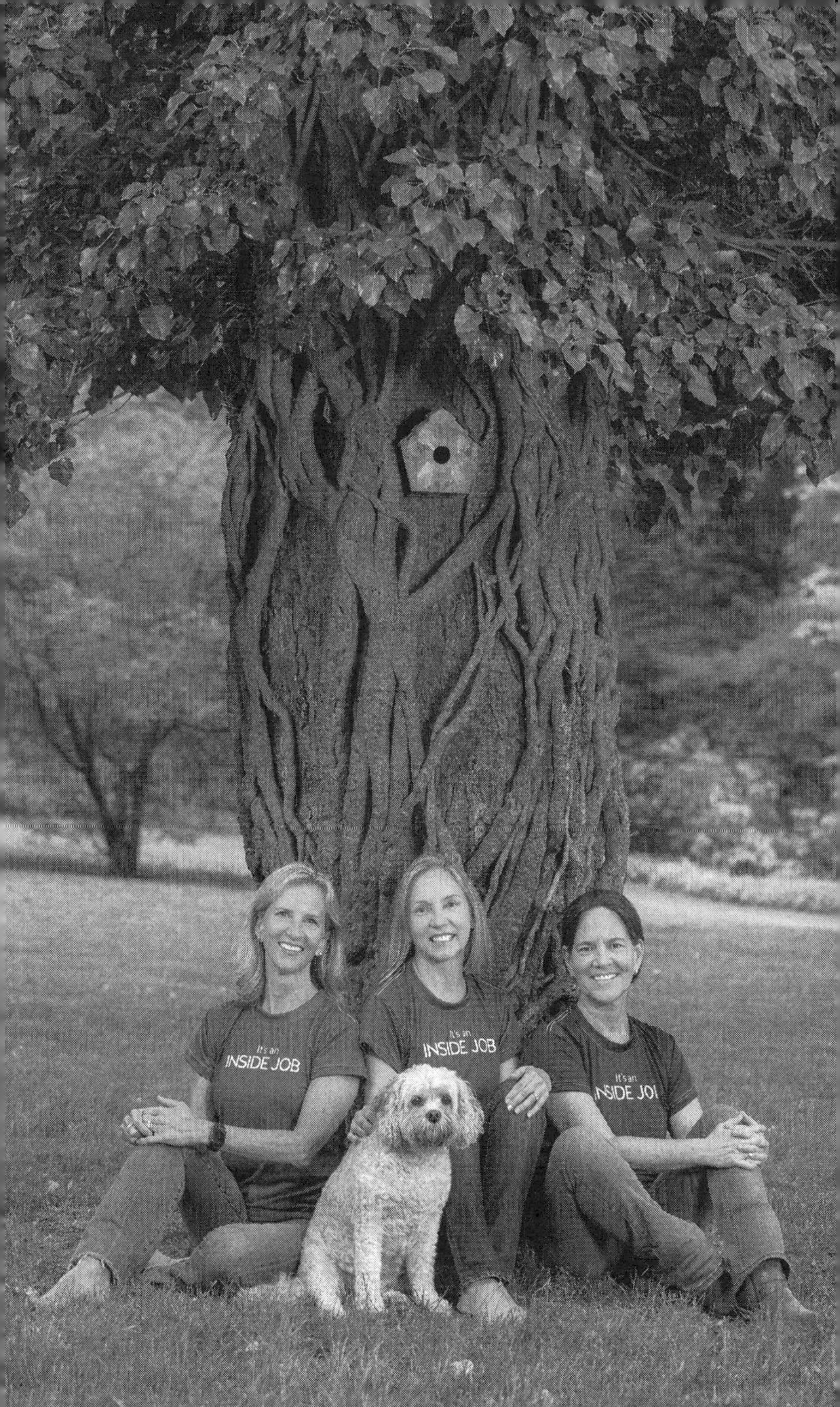
It's an
INSIDE JOB
It's an
INSIDE JOB
It's an
INSIDE JO

Chapter 1

Beginning the Conversation

In the realm of personal growth and self-discovery, the ability to express oneself authentically is akin to turning on a light in the darkest corners of our being. It illuminates the paths we've traveled, unveils the lessons we've learned, and celebrates the resilience that arises from our unique journeys. This authenticity not only enriches our own understanding of ourselves but also resonates with others who may find solace, inspiration, or guidance in our stories.

Never undervalue the freedom we may experience when we begin to make sense to ourselves. Exploring our thoughts, emotions, and experiences enables us to better understand who we are and what matters to us most. As we delve into our inner world and explore the complexities and subtleties of the human experience, we develop greater compassion and understanding for others. We begin the conversation by sharing our unique stories and the defining moments that have shaped us.

Tracy's journey from illness to wellness.

Despite a sunny exterior, I would characterize my younger self as profoundly lonely, heavy-hearted, and unsure of my place in the world. I spent over 20 years attempting to untangle patterns from my youth and fix what seemed broken inside me. Instead of being drawn inward, I spent most of my time seeking solutions outside myself. It is clear the answers I sought were not "out there."

A perfect storm of toxicity manifested into a debilitating illness that was difficult to identify and treat; this compelled me to take control of my life. To help navigate the complexities of the disease, I became my own personal researcher. I attended retreats led by Lyme disease specialists and immersed myself in holistic and natural healing practices. Since the condition was multi-systemic, the wellness strategy needed to be multi-dimensional.

My healing journey opened me up to my inner world. I had to focus on what was happening inside my body, which I honestly had no idea how to inhabit. Long-past traumas and limiting beliefs drove my thoughts and behavior patterns, significantly impacting my life. I discovered that bringing compassion and healing to these places of pain was as vital as eliminating toxins, eradicating pathogens, and supporting my system with proper nutrition.

Focusing on self-care and self-love, I shifted my perspective from "fighting" the illness (and myself) to a more compassionate and gentle one. This change allowed my body to recover from a chronic state of overdrive, giving it a better chance to heal. My new awareness made me realize how crucial it is for all of us to live consciously and seek wellness through a multi-dimensional lens.

Seeing health and wellness as more than physical health is expansive for me. By approaching everything as an experiment, there can be no failure—only successes and lessons learned. I love how nourishing one aspect of life can inspire positive change in another; everything is connected. Conscious living requires mindfulness and intention in all areas of life, from the thoughts we think to the food we eat to the relationships we cultivate and the purpose we foster. As a result, I am creating a more fulfilling and balanced life.

Helping others achieve health and a more profound sense of well-being has become a passion of mine. I hope that sharing our journeys this way makes others feel less alone and inspires them to be brave and vulnerable enough to do their own work. —Tracy

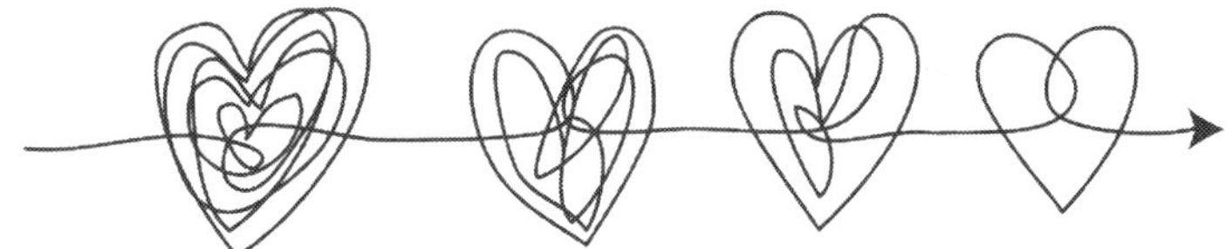

Helen's journey through self-compassion and self-acceptance.

I was 25 years old and pacing my apartment when I caught a glimpse of myself in the mirror. Looking at my reflection, I was hit with an instant moment of truth—I knew the jig was up. I would never outrun my alcoholism. This was my moment of clarity, and it saved my life. I realized I wanted to live more than I wanted to die. So, I laid down my sword, surrendered, and asked God for help. A few days later, I was in treatment.

Even after I became sober, life was still very challenging for me, and I was unconsciously looking outside of myself for solutions. Though my life began to look successful on paper, I was still trying to avoid feeling the pain from my past. My life was ruled by both traumatic events and unconsciously held attachments to outdated beliefs. I felt stuck. I didn't know how to move forward, and there was zero room for self-compassion or self-acceptance—this was my journey.

A significant turning point occurred when I began training in body-centered psychotherapy. I discovered how this therapeutic approach explores the physical body and its manifestations while integrating the mental, physical, and spiritual aspects of who we are. When I started to understand that my body works as a system, I began to allow myself to heal.

By becoming more aware of and developing a deeper understanding of how the body works, I could see that I was unconsciously acting on historical belief patterns. These behaviors no longer served me, yet I often lived them as if they were happening in the present. I learned to feel the pain from my past and move through it thanks to the safety and support I had around me. This is how I opened the door to self-compassion. As a dear mentor often says, "Transformation occurs when one molecule of love meets one molecule of pain."

What I now know for sure is that acceptance requires effort and that healing does not tickle. When we have an open mind and a desire to grow, our journey to self-acceptance is within reach. I now embrace every aspect of my life and use it as a tool to help others. —Helen

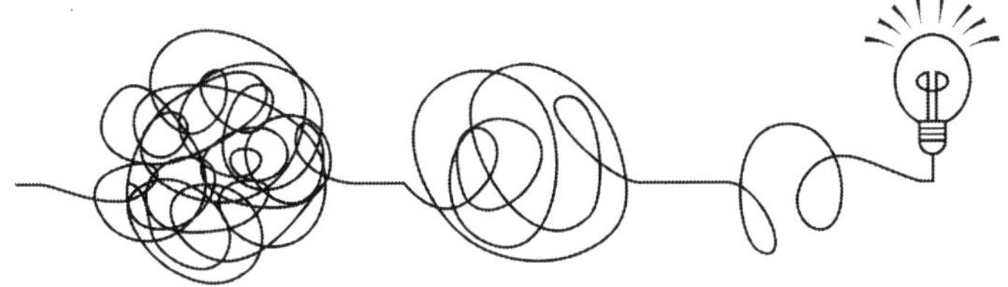

Diane's journey to herself.

Sometimes, I think I woke up at thirty, looked around, and wondered how I got there. My dad only had a few months to live, and I couldn't imagine my life without him; he was my rock. At that point in my life, I was a stay-at-home mom raising three young kids and married to an alcoholic. The drinking was causing emotionally abusive behaviors, and I was living on high alert. My life was exhausting. I wanted it to be less stressful and more joyful.

The following years were spent getting divorced, rebuilding my career, and trying to find myself. I explored various spiritual practices while working 40+ hours a week and attempting to give my children a stable and loving home. It was my intention to discover who I was and what I wanted; however, I never took the time to pause, give myself grace, and accept the magnitude of what I was going through.

Through the years before and since my father's death, my family has experienced a great deal of loss and trauma. One of my earliest life-changing experiences occurred when one of my older brothers was diagnosed with schizophrenia at the age of 18. This diagnosis resulted in both emotional and financial upheaval for my family, particularly during the acute phases of his illness. My sister-in-law tragically passed away, leaving behind two beautiful babies and a gaping hole. It's painful to recall my youngest brother's anguish when his longtime partner and dear friend to all of us died by suicide. Words cannot express the grief we felt when, twice, we had a front-row seat to the devastation that ALS causes. Addiction and alcoholism have taken a toll on our family, and we've also lost loved ones to cancer, dementia, and a literal broken heart. These tragic losses left a lasting impact, forever changing my family dynamics and the way I navigate life.

While I built strength and personal power in my thirties, my healing journey began in my forties. I learned to cry and move some of the emotion that was bottled up inside me from so much loss. Meditation and yoga became a part of my daily routine. I began opening up and having honest conversations with close friends, allowing them to see more of me. Up until then, I kept my life compartmentalized and my feelings contained.

It wasn't until my fifties that I found genuine compassion for myself and the bravery to be more vulnerable; I took the time to dig deeper and got to know myself better from the inside. Now, in my sixties, I live the life I imagined many years ago. I appreciate that the beauty of our journeys can be found in the obstacles put in our way. With the wisdom of making myself a priority, I'm learning how to navigate the world with Jeff, my second husband, who has Parkinson's disease, while also helping an elderly parent give up some of their independence.

Most importantly, I'm learning how to allow myself the space to develop and gain insight from each experience using a multifaceted lens. —Diane

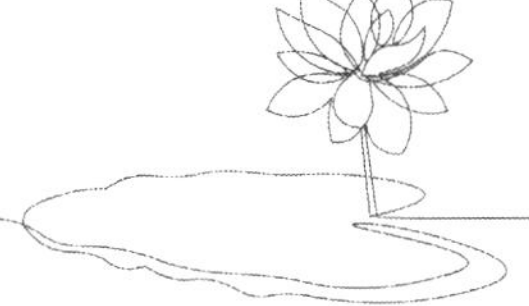

Chapter 2

The Seven Dimensions of Wellness

Your life is calling. It's urging you to push beyond what feels familiar and discover the limitless possibilities inside.

With the rise of chronic illness and mental health issues, there has never been a better time to reclaim your health and wellness, and it starts with seeing and getting to know yourself differently. We want to spark a curiosity that leads to a deeper understanding of YOU. Your relationship with yourself is the most significant one you will ever have. Bringing awareness to your external and internal connections can awaken you to understand yourself better and can lead to a life of greater ease through inspired change.

One of the first steps toward realizing our full potential is learning to love and accept ourselves unconditionally, even the hidden parts of ourselves. Understanding why we do what we do is much easier when we see the body as a system. Our capacity to love and accept ourselves in all our fullness expands when we cultivate self-compassion through mindful living and heightened awareness.

This journey of self-discovery enables us to live authentically and make choices that align with our values and desires. Through this process, we can foster a more profound sense of inner peace and contentment, knowing that we are living in alignment with who we truly are.

We can uncover the layers of our being through curiosity-driven exploration and cultivate a deeper connection with ourselves. It's an inside job. Finding balance and harmony across all aspects of our lives is the key to thriving and flourishing. By nurturing our different dimensions, we can experience a sense of wholeness and fulfillment beyond external achievement, allowing us to live a more joyful and purposeful life.

We are multi-dimensional human beings; our strategy for wellness should be, too!

Thinking of health on a continuum between ease and *dis*-ease can be helpful when planning a wellness journey. This framework was initially conceptualized in 1979 by Dr. Aaron Antonovsky. Between these two states, there can be numerous stressors from various aspects of life, such as poor nutrition, environmental toxins, workplace stress, and unprocessed emotions. Research shows that balance in each dimension is crucial for preserving good health and well-being. We move closer to a life of ease when we can reduce stressors across the spectrum.

When we think about physical fitness as our only health measure without considering our mental well-being, we fall short of what it means to be well; we cannot have physical health without emotional well-being. The World Health Organization (WHO) stated, as early as 1948, that wellness is about striving toward "physical, mental, and social well-being" and is "not merely the absence of disease." In 1976, Dr. Bill Hettler, co-founder of the National Wellness Institute (NWI), identified Six Dimensions of Wellness to help build a holistic sense of harmony and fulfillment. Environmental health has been added to the list, making it a comprehensive list of seven dimensions that are interconnected and interwoven.

By identifying and bringing balance where needed, we can incorporate a shift in mindset, wellness-affirming rituals, and more self-love into our daily practices. Since all the dimensions are interconnected, one is not more significant than the others. However, because caring for our mind is the most crucial preventative health measure and how we create our lives, this book begins with understanding and caring for it. First, let's begin with a brief description of each element of wellness:

Intellectual wellness is being curious, open to differing views, and willing to challenge everything we think we know. It also means being aware of our power to create.

Emotional wellness is understanding ourselves and embracing life's challenges; it is acknowledging, accepting, and sharing feelings of anger, fear, sadness, distress, hope, love, joy, and happiness.

Social wellness means establishing and nurturing positive relationships with self, family, friends, and co-workers while maintaining healthy boundaries. It is realizing every relationship is impacted by how we feel about ourselves.

Environmental wellness is being in tune with how our everyday life impacts us and taking responsibility for what we're exposed to in our homes, work, relationships, and greater surroundings. It is being aware of how our environment affects us and, in turn, how we affect the environment.

Occupational wellness is gaining personal fulfillment from a job, career, or volunteer position while maintaining balance.

Spiritual wellness is our most profound level of consciousness. It is being connected to something greater than ourselves and finding meaning and purpose in life.

Physical wellness means listening to the body as a guide while nourishing and taking care of it for optimal health and functioning.

Starting from wherever you are, you can create the life you desire by taking responsibility for all the dimensions of your life. Most wellness paradigms suggest that the physical dimension is the cornerstone of general wellness. Instead, we identify with Dr. Lissa Rankin's health cairn, where the physical dimension sits on top. Dr. Rankin is a mind-body medicine physician and founder of the Whole Health Medicine Institute. She believes physical health will always be essential, but foundationally, the body does not need to be in peak condition to have meaningful relationships or a successful career. Instead, she encourages us to consider the body a barometer for wellness in other dimensions; it lets us know when our lives become unhealthy or out of alignment.

> Like a car's dashboard lights, our body uses signals to communicate when something is out of alignment with our true self. Deciphering our body's messages requires a deeper understanding of it.

Silos are a part of our culture; we see them in our workplaces, healthcare system, and society. Nothing thrives when the focus is on separate parts of the system. Instead, the emphasis should be on the interconnectedness of all the parts of the whole. A holistic approach to wellness means looking at the whole person through each interconnected dimension, being evermore curious about what is happening in and around us, and understanding our stories compassionately. Discovering that we are shaping our futures, knowingly or not, is life-changing. Even though it may not feel that way right now, we are each the creators of our stories.

Before we go on to each of the seven dimensions, we'd like to encourage a new way of thinking about ourselves. It is pivotal to see the body as an operating system rather than identify with our heightened emotions, thoughts, circumstances, or patterns. We believe that gaining knowledge about the nervous system will lead to a deeper understanding of who we are. Stay with us because we need to get a little scientific in order to explain!

Human Nervous System

CENTRAL NERVOUS SYSTEM
(The body's master control unit)

The CNS consists of the brain and the spinal cord. It is responsible for processing and coordinating information received from the sensory organs and sending signals to different parts of the body.

PERIPHERAL NERVOUS SYSTEM
(the body's link to the outside world)

The PNS consists of nerves that branch out from your CNS throughout your entire body, and it relays information from your brain and spinal cord, from your organs to your fingers and toes

Somatic Nervous System

The SNS controls voluntary movements like walking and talking, and it carries sensory information like touch, temperature, and pain to the CNS.

Autonomic Nervous System

Operating automatically without conscious direction, the ANS regulates involuntary processes including heart rate, breathing, and digestion.

Sympathetic Nervous System

Responsible for "fight or flight" response; prepares the body for action. Increases heart rate, dilates blood vessels and releases adrenaline.

Parasympathetic Nervous System

Promotes relaxation and conserves energy. It slows down heart rate, constricts blood vessels, and aids in digestion and elimination.

Vagus nerve

Relied on by the parasympathetic nervous system to control heart rate, respiration, and digestion. Reduces "fight or flight" reaction to stress, promoting feelings of calm and relaxation, as well as supporting social engagement and connection.

Let's go inside!

Everything is energy, and our system functions like an antenna, picking up and transmitting information to every part of our body. We experience and respond to life through our nervous system; the body is the first to inform us of our surroundings and helps us navigate through the world. Although essential to human survival, this complex network doesn't get enough attention when discussing health and wellness.

Why is it important to become friends with our nervous system? Being curious about this system allows us to see better not only how we are but who we are. It's like checking in on a good friend who is always there but often goes unnoticed. Understanding the nervous system is crucial because it governs our thoughts, emotions, and behaviors; it helps us understand why we do what we do. By developing a friendship with it, we can gain insights into the intricate workings of our mind and body, leading to improved self-awareness, self-care, and personal growth. When we have a deeper understanding of how our nervous system responds to different situations, we can learn to identify and address triggers more effectively, leading to a greater sense of calm and overall well-being.

What happens in Vagus? We know people don't like to talk about what happens in Vegas, but the vagus nerve can't stop talking; it's our body's communication superhighway. This remarkable nerve is the longest cranial nerve, running from the brain to the large intestine (think mind-body connection!). Vagus nerve function contributes to our autonomic system and regulates heart rate, breathing, and digestion. When stressed, this nerve helps return us to a state of calm. Chronic stress, however, can lead to a weakened vagus nerve, which can result in physical responses such as digestive issues, inflammation, and even depression. Therefore, keeping it healthy and functioning properly is crucial for overall well-being.

When we consider the body as a system, we can better understand that it is built to defend itself; it puts safety above everything. When our nervous system detects a potential threat, real or imagined, it triggers the fight-or-flight response to ensure our survival.

> *"To be "well" is not to live in a state of perpetual safety and calm, but to move fluidly from a state of adversity, risk, adventure, or excitement, back to safety and calm, and out again. Stress is not bad for you; being stuck is bad for you."*
>
> —Emily Nagoski

A healthy nervous system moves back and forth between states of activation and relaxation. This provides rhythm, balance, and harmony for all bodily functions the ANS governs. Understanding these responses can help us determine what motivates us to act and how to manage our stress levels better.

Safe and Connected (parasympathetic state). We move into a state of flow when the nervous system detects safety. These are the feelings Dorothy from *The Wizard of Oz* longed for when she said, "There's no place like home." This feeling of being at home is not limited to a physical location; it is a state of mind that allows us to be ourselves and fosters a sense of belonging in our bodies and the world around us. Here, we might experience a sense of peace and contentment where we can tap into our creativity, intuition, and inner wisdom. This state is also known as "rest and digest," where our bodies can relax, heal, and rejuvenate. In this state, our digestion improves, our immune system strengthens, and our overall well-being is enhanced. It is essential to cultivate this state regularly to maintain a healthy balance in our lives and foster a deep connection with ourselves and those around us. Our goal isn't to remain here; calm isn't always fitting. However, we want to come back here often.

On Alert (sympathetic state). When the body senses a threat, it mobilizes us. This protective state is better known as "fight-or-flight," where our body assesses real or perceived danger. In this state, our heart rate increases, our muscles tense, and our focus narrows as we prepare to either confront the threat or run away from it. This heightened state of alertness can be helpful in certain situations, but if we remain in this state for too long, it can lead to chronic stress and burnout. It is essential to find ways to calm ourselves down and return to a more relaxed state to maintain overall well-being.

We are taught to believe stress is harmful—"stress will kill us." Is this true? In the short term, stress can leave us anxious and struggling to cope, but if that stress becomes chronic or, for instance, a two thousand-pound bull is chasing us on the streets of Barcelona, we might be in trouble. However, the effect of stress most often depends on our frame of mind.

What if we practice seeing non-life-threatening stress as a motivator or an agent of change? According to Dr. Kelly McGonigal, health psychologist and lecturer at Stanford University, stress can build resiliency, boost cognitive function, and act as a powerful motivator if we learn to use it to our advantage. While it takes some practice, it is possible to train our brains to see stress as a helpful tool; this is called a growth mindset. So, try not to stress over stress! Only in utopia would we live uninterrupted in a safe and connected state; we joke about how boring it would be if we were always there. Okay, so a little more often would be terrific! That's the goal.

Shut Down and Freeze (sympathetic state). If the nervous system senses that the bull is gaining on us or we are completely overwhelmed by our situation, it will move us into Shut Down or Freeze. In the wilderness, this is where animals "play dead" in a last-ditch effort to save themselves. In humans, this may sometimes look like 'laziness' or anti-social behavior creating unfair judgment, when Shut Down is a mode of disconnection for self-preservation. This immobilized state is the body's way of protecting itself. However, if an individual remains here for prolonged periods, it can have detrimental effects on their physical and mental well-being.

The good news is that these responses are all needed, normal, and meant to be temporary. The nervous system is designed to protect us; it senses what is happening in and around us, shares that information with the brain, and moves us to act accordingly. Remember, though, that much of this occurs without our awareness. Be curious; there's so much to learn about why we do what we do. We can't reach our full potential for growth and connection from a dysregulated or weakened nervous system.

We want to experience all that life has to offer, including risk, adventure, and excitement, rather than always being at "home." Observing a dog on a walk is an excellent way to witness the flow between states. Watch as the dog happily trots along. Suddenly, in response to a real or perceived threat, the dog's gait will change, and the hair on its neck will stand up. Then, when the dog feels safe again, the fur will fall, and the gait will return to a trot. This movement between states happens countless times as the dog senses and evaluates its environment. Imagine similar shifts occurring repeatedly in your body.

Even though our system is perfectly designed for us, modern life moves so quickly that we don't often notice how long we've been away from the safety and security of "home." We may distract ourselves with junk food, social media, addictive substances, and other self-destructive behaviors to avoid the messages of imbalance our body is sending. Many of us seek treatment from the doctor for pain management when we are going through something entirely different on the inside. It's important to note studies show 80% of our thoughts are negative, and 95% of them are repetitive. So, imagine what can happen to our nervous system when we become attached to some of those adverse thoughts.

DYSREGULATION: Sometimes, we do get stuck!

When the nervous system is exposed to continuous stress in one or more of our dimensions, the natural flow between states can become disrupted. Factors like emotional wounds, a buildup of environmental toxins, physical stress, dietary factors, and workplace or relationship stress can all contribute to dysregulation. Ruminating on negative thoughts can further exacerbate the situation; imagine what a worldwide pandemic and political unrest can do! When we start spending too much time in a stressed or immobilized state, we can get stuck there.

When our body's internal control breaks down, it can misinterpret what's going on around it, sending the wrong messages to our brain. Because of this, it may become harder to keep our feelings and behaviors in check. Being in a state of "fight, flight, freeze or collapse" for long periods can have many negative effects on our body and mind, including stress, anxiety, sadness, digestive issues, high blood pressure, and a weaker immune system. Not being able to return to the parasympathetic state can have an adverse effect on every aspect of our lives.

Let's use the example of a person who experiences chronic stress at work. This individual may constantly feel on edge, continually anticipating threats or challenges. Their body remains in a state of heightened alertness, with an increased heart rate and elevated cortisol levels. This prolonged sympathetic nervous system activation can eventually affect their physical health, leading to chronic fatigue, muscle tension, and cardiovascular problems. Additionally, their mental well-being may suffer as they struggle to find a sense of calm and relaxation outside of work, impacting their relationships and overall quality of life. The bottom line is that when our nervous system is out of sync, so are we! Because humans are resilient, we can regain our equilibrium by slowing down, changing our environment, or seeking support from a trusted friend or therapist. In a later chapter, we offer our favorite practices for nourishing the vagus nerve, the conduit that leads you "home" to safety and connection.

The body remembers: Like every biological process, the stress cycle has a beginning, middle, and end. When we experience something that overwhelms us, we often cannot complete the cycle, and the responding energy remains stored in the body. A current event can trigger a memory, and the body will react to protect us as if it were happening here and now. So, even if you're safe in the present moment, your system may communicate that trauma energy is still there, waiting to be discharged. Think of triggers as flashing lights indicating that something inside needs attention and tending to.

You make perfect sense!

When we take the time to pause and recognize what is happening inside, it allows for more compassion for where we are. The biggest takeaway from learning more about our internal workings is that there is nothing wrong with us; our system functions as it was designed. Building resources and a sense of trust and safety are essential for navigating life. It's impossible to find our YES! from a state of fight, flight, or freeze. Grounding ourselves and accessing that safety in the present moment allows us to move through our struggles more easily.

In the coming chapters, we will share encouraging stories of overcoming life's difficulties. We can learn more about ourselves and our place in the world by exploring the seven interconnected yet distinct facets of who we are. When we examine these dimensions and look to heal or grow forward, the message to the body needs to be one of safety and connection. Then, as we practice embracing our vulnerabilities and sharing our experiences, we can foster compassion, allowing us to support one another meaningfully.

In our search for greater ease, we have found that happiness is not a destination but a state of mind. Being in the now and finding delight in the little things are essential to life's journey. Later in the book, we share the heartbreaking story of Tracy's sister Leigh, who tragically loses her house in a wildfire yet manages to find moments of light and comfort in a chance encounter with a llama. So that our pain does not consume us, we cling to these moments. Despite the imperfections and chaos of life, there is always a hint of hope or a moment of joy.

> Search for the glimmers. The sparkles. The fireflies. By collecting all of these pieces of gold along the way, we create a deep, meaningful, and rich existence.

There is a duality to life in our struggles and joys. Embracing both the light and the dark allows us to appreciate the beauty in every moment. In bringing awareness to and embracing the wholeness of who we are, we discover our true selves and what deeply matters to us. As we embark on this journey of self-discovery and explore our seven dimensions, we aim to spark curiosity and inspire others to live more intentionally, meaningfully, and compassionately.

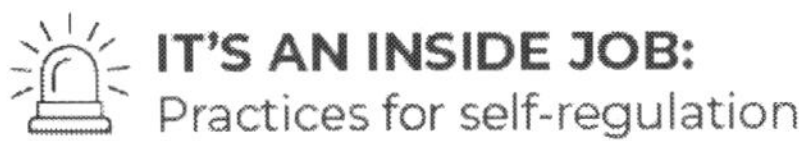

When our nervous system is healthy, we can effortlessly transition between stimulation and safety. The key to adaptability in life is the capacity to better manage our emotions. Having the skills to self-regulate is essential for maintaining balance across the dimensions of wellness.

Hit the Pause Button

We all know how easy it is to react impulsively after an experience has disturbed our state of calm. As described in an article for Well+Good, Neuroscientist and mental-health specialist Caroline Leaf, Ph.D., says that after an event, there will be an initial biochemical and electrical spike lasting 30 to 90 seconds where our unconscious and conscious mind adapts and digests the incoming information. This short time frame is where we tend to act without thinking.

Instead of responding immediately, try practicing the Pause to help your system return to a state of safety and connection. Take a deep breath, expand your rib cage on the inhale, and then focus on a strong exhale. Repeat three to five times. This practice helps to send a message of "I'm safe!" to your body while creating space between you and the event. If needed, change your location or do something physical to move the energy in your body. The idea is to allow at least 30 to 90 seconds to pass, creating the opportunity for a thoughtful response versus a spontaneous reaction.

Self-Talk Is Powerful

As we become aware of how many negative thoughts the mind produces, we can consciously avoid attaching to those thoughts in challenging situations. One of the ways to do this is by asking yourself questions like, "What is one good thing about this situation?" "What can I learn from this challenge?" or "How would my best friend support me?"

Dr. Judy Ho, a licensed and triple board-certified clinical and forensic neuropsychologist, recommends singing negative thoughts to an upbeat song. For instance, sing "Today is going to be the most stressful day" to the tune Happy Birthday. "You'll notice that it takes the air out of the negative thought, and you are more likely to take less stock in the doom and gloom thoughts that will further deregulate your nervous system," she says.

Befriend the Resistance

Bringing in a bit of playfulness is fun and beneficial. When you're becoming aware of your negative thought patterns and stories in stressful situations, personify them like they are your friends.

"Oh, hey, Worry! I see you there."

"Hello, Doubt! Welcome to the conversation."

Then, attach a growth mindset response as this becomes more comfortable. "Oh, hey, Worry! I see you, but there's no reason for concern. All Clear." "Hello, Doubt. Welcome to the conversation. Step aside and watch me do this!"

Personifying them helps to avoid getting caught in the thought spiral. Practicing with a growth mindset can help you self-regulate in stressful situations, allowing you more ease.

Use Your YES!

So many of us are disconnected from our bodies; we've lost the ability to feel. One of the most effective ways to start practicing somatic (bodily) awareness is from a state of safety and connection. When something is for us, our body sends the message of YES! through an energetic resonance. Keeping a YES! journal brings awareness to our sensations and reminds us of all that is for us.

Start by recording experiences, activities, sensations, and insights that speak YES! to you. Seeing and recording the good in each day illuminates what resonates deep within you. With discernment, learning to trust that feeling of YES! is like a guiding light; these pages will start to paint a picture of what lights your soul on fire.

It may be surprising to learn that journaling is considered one of the best wellness tools. It can put space between you and negative thoughts, give you clarity, encourage you to let go, and help you bring some of your deepest desires to life.

Just Breathe

It sounds almost too easy, but simple breathing exercises can bring calm to your system. We use the 4-4-4-4 box breathing recommended by Dr. Judy Ho. Inhale on a count of four, hold for four counts, exhale for four counts, and hold for four counts. Then, repeat for a total of 10 rounds. Visualizing your way around a box can be helpful.

Intellectual

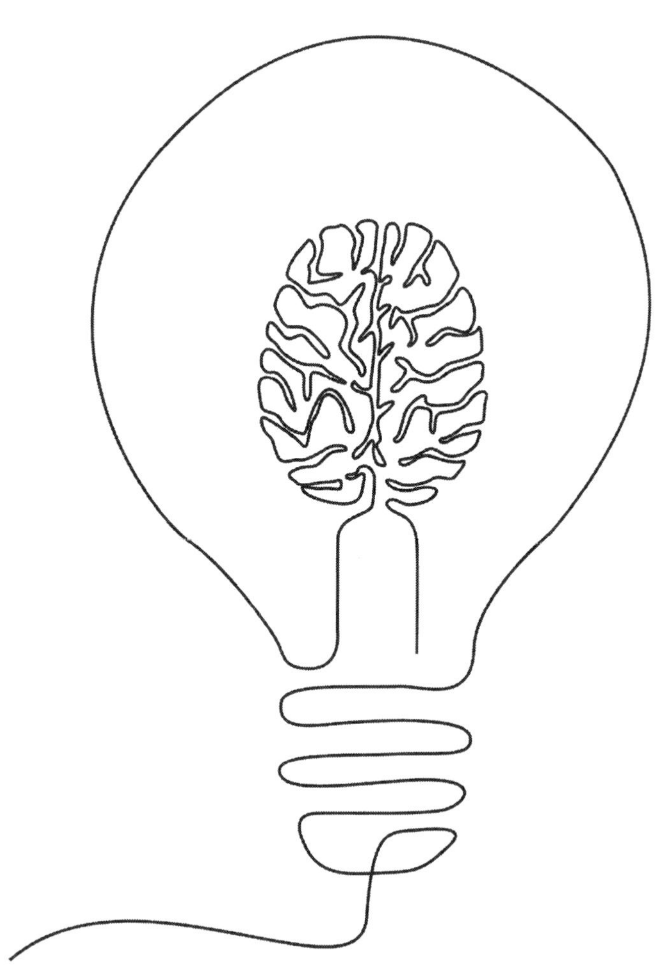

I am curious,
aware, and always
learning—I have the
power to create.

“Curiosity. Millions saw the apple fall, but Newton asked why.”

—Bernard Baruch

Chapter 3

Intellectual Wellness

We ask why a lot when we are young. We see the world around us and want to know more; we want to understand. At what age do you think most people start becoming less curious? Intellectual wellness is not about how smart we are, what our IQ is, or where and if we went to college; it is about a never-ending curiosity and willingness to learn. A lifelong learner stays open to exploring new topics and is never afraid to ask why.

We may try new things, read books, take classes, and engage in hobbies to strengthen this dimension, but we often ignore the one thing that has the most significant influence on our health and happiness. We tend to study everything but ourselves! Research shows that curiosity can impact our emotional, psychological, physical, and social health. So, by picking up this book to read, you have already demonstrated that you are curious and want to learn more about your personal power.

Intellectual wellness is being curious, open to differing views, and willing to challenge everything you think you know. It also means being aware of your power to create.

Let's begin our discussion of this dimension with some fun facts about the brain. This complex organ comprises about 2% of the body's total weight but uses 20% of its energy and oxygen intake. Weighing nearly three pounds, it's the fattiest organ in the body. Despite what we've been told about avoiding fat, cholesterol (HDL—the good kind) is an integral part of every brain cell; without an adequate supply, those cells die. Proper nourishment, including a whole-food diet rich in vitamins and healthy fats, hydration, and exercise, is essential for healthy brain function.

The brain is 73% water, and even the slightest bit of dehydration affects attention, memory, and other cognitive skills. Drinking water first thing in the morning can help replenish the body's water levels after an overnight fast. Try an experiment for 30 days by drinking 8–16 ounces of water upon waking (before coffee and food!). Bonus points if you add a squeeze of lemon. Be aware of any subtle changes.

We are surprised to learn the most advanced computers are no match for the human brain. This fact ups our swagger a bit; we must be something! Then, we are reminded that 95% of our thoughts and decisions occur in the subconscious mind; suddenly, we realize we're not so in control. The brain stores a lifetime of experiences, beliefs, emotions, memories, dreams, motivations, and habits, and our subconscious mind draws on them to make decisions.

According to Dr. Joe Dispenza, neuroscientist, and researcher, "95% of who we are by the time we're 35 years old is a memorized set of behaviors, emotional reactions, unconscious habits, hardwired attitudes, beliefs, and perceptions that function like a computer program."

Think about it this way: we learn about the world from our earliest surroundings and those who raised us. Our worldview is shaped by what we were exposed to and conditioned to believe. What motivates us today may be tied to our earliest perceptions, even if they no longer align with who we've become as autonomous adults. We live in a fast-paced society where we don't take the time to understand why we keep repeating specific negative patterns despite having positive goals and desires. We look for answers outside ourselves when we feel stuck or believe something is missing.

By bringing curiosity to our thoughts and behaviors, we can uncover the underlying beliefs and conditioning that drive our actions. This self-awareness allows us to make conscious choices and break free from the limitations of our past. It empowers us to create a new narrative that aligns with the future we wish to create.

The power of the mind—manifestation in action.

With an inquisitive lens, let's revisit the idea that our thoughts shape our reality. This is not a mystical concept but the science of how we function; we are what we think. We choose our thoughts, our thoughts inform our actions, and our actions create our reality. Therefore, it is important to cultivate positive and empowering thoughts to shape a positive and empowering life.

When we realize we have a conscious choice, we see that we have the power to create.

Conscious choice is our superpower. However, it is critical to remember that the only way to make a conscious choice is in the here and now. Otherwise, the subconscious decides for us based on stored information. This is why mindfulness practices, such as meditation and deep breathing, can be so powerful in helping us become more present and aware. As we quiet the chatter of our minds, we can make intentional decisions and shape our own narrative.

Of course, many aspects of life are beyond our control, and we cannot change them even from a place of awareness. The silver lining? We always have the power to choose our response. Let's take a breakup, for example. If your default response over time is, "He left me, and I'll never find love again," you might feel lost or stuck in the cycle of sadness and despair, finding it difficult to move on.

Instead, if your response is, "I feel so sad, but if I'm not valued, I need to find someone who loves and appreciates me," you're more likely to treat yourself right and look for new opportunities. Now, don't get us wrong—it doesn't mean moving on is easy or that you won't feel sadness. It's about allowing yourself to feel the pain and then choosing to take steps towards healing and growth. By choosing a response that empowers you, you can navigate through the hurt and eventually find happiness again. Essentially, you change your future trajectory by how you respond.

"Okay, so being able to influence our lives seems plausible; why isn't creating the life we want easier?" Often, it's because the mind has a mind of its own. This concept highlights the complex and dynamic nature of human cognition and consciousness. Remember, the mind is a system, and the subconscious draws from a database filled with a memorized set of behaviors, emotional reactions, unconscious habits, hardwired attitudes, views, and perceptions. These ingrained patterns of thinking and behaving can often hinder our ability to manifest the life we desire.

Don't always believe what your mind tells you.

One of the most critical signs of development in this dimension is recognizing the mind as a thought generator. Have you noticed that it talks incessantly? Eckhart Tolle believes we should not identify with our thoughts but rather observe them. Using this perspective, we can learn to witness our thoughts without getting caught up in them and make better decisions based on our values and goals.

Remember, the mind doesn't force us to accept its ideas; it simply makes suggestions. With conscious awareness, we can choose to accept or reject the thoughts that arise in our minds. This empowers us to align our actions with our true desires and intentions rather than being controlled by the constant chatter.

Intellectual wellness means pausing to ask ourselves, "Why am I thinking this?" "Is this true?" or "Is this a story my mind is generating based on an experience or limiting belief?" and then choosing our next thought. We begin to reprogram our subconscious mind by replacing negative thoughts and historical beliefs with thinking that aligns with our goals. Then, by reinforcing these thoughts, they become our new default mode of thinking. Although it requires practice, this gives us a great deal of creative control.

"When you make a choice, you change the future."
—Deepak Chopra

Are you starting to realize how much power you have? The mind gives credibility to repeated positive or negative thoughts and converts them into beliefs. We use this lens as a filter when looking for evidence to support our reasoning. By consciously choosing positive and empowering thoughts, we can reprogram our minds to filter for evidence that supports our growth and success. This, in turn, helps us make choices aligning with our highest potential and purpose.

If you start to see negative patterns, it may be time to look deeper to identify a limiting belief. We can break out of unfavorable thought patterns and make decisions more consistent with our goals and values by identifying and challenging or healing what might be holding us back on the inside.

How our system reinforces our limiting beliefs.

We think it's remarkable how the brain will look for whatever our subconscious mind tells it to find. Have you ever noticed that after learning something new, you encounter it everywhere? This type of experience is called the Baader-Meinhof phenomenon, also known as the frequency illusion or frequency bias.

This phenomenon can have both positive and negative effects on our lives. On the one hand, it can help us learn and grow by exposing us to new information, but it can also lead to confirmation bias, where the brain searches for information that supports a current belief or value we hold. This means our brains look to reinforce what we already believe.

For example, if our friend, Sue, wants to be a successful artist, her brain will seek out information about herself as an artist. However, if Sue's inner dialogue is full of doubts and thoughts that she isn't talented enough, she will find proof that she isn't skilled as an artist. The brain finds information to support a belief, and Sue believes she isn't enough.

Reaching our goals may be impossible if something formidable holds us back on the inside. We can't be worthy and unworthy at the same time. Good news! The opposite is also true. If our thoughts are consistent with our goals and aspirations and we surround ourselves with people who believe in us, we will continue to discover our worth. The mind is a system that can either empower us or limit us! Therefore, it is crucial to cultivate a positive mindset and surround ourselves with supportive people who encourage us to reach our full potential.

"If you find a path with no obstacles, it probably doesn't lead anywhere." —Frank A. Clark

"How do I transform these limiting beliefs into positive ones?" The first step is becoming aware of the core convictions you hold. You can do this by listening. As we've mentioned, the mind is a thought generator; it talks incessantly. According to the Laboratory of Neuro Imaging at the University of Southern California, the mind gives rise to 48.6 thoughts per minute or 70,000 daily. It is impossible to police all of our thoughts, but becoming more aware of our patterns is an essential move toward changing these beliefs. As with any change, awareness is the first step.

Once you've identified a belief such as "I'm not good enough," try to connect with where it originated. Is it true, or did someone in the past make you feel that way? For example, imagine if Sue made the connection to her fourth-grade art teacher, who told her she would never be an artist.

This experience has no bearing on Sue as an artist today, but her outdated subconscious belief system is holding her back. Sue can create new pathways by compassionately meeting her fourth-grade self and reframing the experience with a new perspective that empowers her as an artist today. This technique is called inner-child work and can be a powerful tool for personal growth and healing.

Through this lens, Helen had little trouble making the connections to her childhood that led to her most damaging beliefs. Studies show there is a strong link between traumatic childhood experiences and addictive behaviors in adulthood. Healing the perceptions she held tightly in her youth helped her become the confident and inspiring woman she is today. Helen's experiences and perseverance fueled her desire to get her master's in therapy and addiction counseling.

"I grew up in the '70s and '80s, and in that era, there was little acceptance of homosexuals in my community and among some of my family members. I often witnessed gay people taking the brunt of bad 'jokes' or being the target of hostile encounters. As a young teenager, I was on the wrong side of cultural norms when I realized I was gay. While I had a small number of people I felt comfortable being "me" around, being rejected by the people I loved the most set me on a lengthy path of self-destruction.

After getting sober, my therapist suggested I imagine how I saw myself from the inside and create a visual. The idea was to design something tactile so I could see it. For me, the split within myself showed up as four separate and distinct bricks:

— *Who I was with my immediate family.*
— *Who I was at work.*
— *Who I was with my straight friends, some of whom were homophobic.*
— *Who I was with my gay friends.*

The bricks represented how I needed to suit up for the day. I was often in a state of fight-or-flight; which brick did I have to be? I was constantly expecting the worst-case scenario—which for me was someone finding out who I was. My life had become compartmentalized, and I wore very different masks; the insides of those masks were dark and empty. Internalized homophobia tormented me. It was terrifying, confusing, and exhausting.

Working with a professional was vital for my healing. I found somatic therapy to be extremely enriching for me; the body is the foundation for heal-

ing in this modality. Understanding that my implicit memories remained trapped inside my body, I've been able to meet the pain I held onto for many years—and drop into the grief that is underneath the anger—that resulted from not being loved for who I am.

Healing is hard work—it doesn't tickle—but I am so grateful. I no longer need to separate from myself or wear masks; I am most comfortable being myself. Along with my practice and continuing my education to help others, maintaining a growth mindset is of utmost importance for my well-being."

"Becoming is better than being." —Carol Dweck

A growth mindset is one of this dimension's most important indicators for optimal health. Carol Dweck, a Stanford University psychologist, found people are influenced by two perspectives—growth and fixed. A growth mindset reveals a love of learning and the belief that skills like intelligence and creativity, as well as qualities like love and friendship, can be developed and improved with commitment and hard work. This mental expansion also promotes self-regulation by teaching us to value struggle, obstacles, fear, mistakes, and failures.

In contrast, a fixed mindset is a belief system in which individuals believe that their abilities, intelligence, and qualities are mainly static and unchangeable. A fixed perspective resists change and is a self-perpetuating obstacle that can prevent people from reaching their potential in every dimension. Individuals with a fixed mindset may shy away from situations where they might not immediately excel because they fear failure, which they perceive as a reflection of their inherent abilities. It can be challenging to recognize this belief system in ourselves, as it often operates unconsciously. However, reflecting on our reactions to challenges and setbacks can provide insight.

Characteristics of a Growth Mindset:

— I am always capable of growing and improving no matter the obstacle.
— My comfort zone shows me where I can expand.
— I know mistakes are part of the learning process.
— I am willing to take on challenges with determination.
— I am open to feedback and willing to learn from it.
— I believe failures are chances to learn.
— I celebrate the successes of myself and others, no matter how small.
— I am worthy of happiness and love.
— If I find myself in judgment of others, I know there is inner work to do.
— I take personal responsibility for my actions.
— I embrace strength in community and teamwork.
— I focus on and enjoy the journey, not just the destination.

Characteristics of a Fixed Mindset:

x I am who I am.
x I am happy in my comfort zone.
x I see mistakes as personal flaws.
x I avoid challenges for fear of failure.
x I take criticism personally.
x I feel threatened by the success of others.
x I give up when the going gets tough.
x I judge and label others.
x I make excuses or blame others.
x I cannot be on a team without being in charge.
x I miss the journey by getting hung up on results.

It's easy to grasp how anything is possible with a growth mindset; it is an excellent practice and can help bring us back to a safe and connected state where we can reach for the stars. Most of us have a combination of mindsets; no doubt, each of us can find ourselves in at least one of those fixed examples.

Curiosity can help us connect a fixed mindset characteristic to a limiting belief, just like the artist who kept finding reasons to doubt herself. But it's important to remember that the source of those limiting thoughts is stored in the body, and it can't always be "fixed" because the mind decides it is so. Often, limiting beliefs come from experiences that were too painful for us to deal with at the time. Returning to the body in the present, bringing compassion to ourselves, and working to move the stuck energy can bring deep release and transformation.

Dysregulation may drive negative beliefs. The health of our nervous system has a significant impact on how we think. We can't use the regions of our brain responsible for new and creative thinking when we're in "fight-or-flight" or "freeze" mode. When the neurological system is out of balance, it can cause negative thinking patterns and biases, which can impair a person's behavior and decision-making capacity. As a result, creating a supportive and encouraging atmosphere can help us feel secure and connected. It is important to prioritize a healthy nervous system for optimal cognitive performance.

How do I develop a growth mindset?

Developing a growth mindset can help us embrace challenges, learn from failures, and ultimately grow and improve in various aspects of our lives. Remember, it must be an ongoing practice to have a significant impact on our personal development. Over time, it can help us become more adaptable, resilient, and open to new opportunities.

Here are some simple tips to put into practice the next time you face a challenge. Try using these exercises to help you shift from a *fixed* perspective to a *growth mindset*:

Be courageous. There will always be adversities, but taking a moment to redefine the circumstance as an "opportunity" changes how we consider things. Adopt the motto "There are no failures, only opportunities to learn and grow."

Be mindful. Positive reflections should take the place of negative ones. Saying "I can't do this," for instance, should be changed to "I can't do this, YET." Practice bringing encouragement and compassion to yourself.

Be open to feedback. Friends, family, and co-workers may observe what you are doing from a different angle and offer some useful advice. Seek guidance with the knowledge that the ultimate choice is yours. Trust yourself while being open to others.

Learn from others. No one needs to go it alone. Learning from the successes or missteps of others can help you reach your goal with more ease. Knowing someone has tried before can also calm the fear of tackling this opportunity. Other people's attitudes and beliefs can be contagious and provide support and inspiration for your own growth journey.

Embrace challenges. Instead of avoiding challenges or tasks that may be difficult, embrace them. View challenges as opportunities for learning and growth. When you encounter a difficult task, remind yourself that it's a chance to develop new skills and knowledge.

Keep it real. Rewiring your brain takes time. Remember, the outcome is less important when you adopt a growth mindset. You can always begin again. The more you invest in your growth, the more you can achieve.

Anyone who wants to develop a growth mindset can do so with practice.

We can train our minds to work for us and increase our chances of creating the results we want. A gratitude practice can impact our mindset and transform our lives. Thoughts, words, and actions can be influential but not as powerful as when we fuel them with emotion. Did you know one of the strongest human emotions is gratitude?

"When some things go wrong, take a moment to be thankful for the many things that are going right.
—Annie Gottlier

Cultivating this positive emotion can be as easy as generating five things you're thankful for before closing your eyes each night. Another suggestion is to keep a journal of the little things you experience throughout the day that give you a "Yes!" resonance. Or start a gratitude jar. Keep a pen and small pieces of paper beside a container and add notes of gratitude daily. Then, read them for a pick-me-up when feeling down.

Tracy's gratitude ritual goes beyond keeping a Yes! journal and helps everyone in the house start the day with joy. She chooses to jump out of bed each morning with an exclamation of gratitude. For example, one day, as soon as her feet touch the floor, she might throw her hands in the air and yell, "Yes! I'm alive!" The following day, she may leap out of bed and exclaim, "Good morning, world! Today is a great day!"

Although this amusing custom started as an experiment to see if it affected her mindset (it did!), she continues doing it because it also brings joy to anyone in hearing distance. Who doesn't want to laugh a little to start the day? Being thankful for what you have or living from a place of abundance means the brain will be searching for more of the same. Starting the day with a positive mindset and expressing gratitude sets the tone for a day filled with positivity and opportunities.

The brain is the system; the mind helps to shape our biology.

It is a bold assertion to claim that the mind can impact the physical body. We don't want to become locked in the ego, believing that the conscious mind is all-powerful since the conscious mind isn't always in control. Yet, magic occurs when our ideas, actions, and related unconscious beliefs are in harmony. We have historically been told we are victims of our genes. So, if a disease or health condition like heart disease, cancer, or diabetes runs in the family, we tend to think that our genes decide our fate. However, many scientists believe that our genes change and react to our environment. This means that everything we think, do, say, eat, drink, experience, or hold in our bodies can affect our biology.

Ovarian cancer ranks fifth in cancer deaths among women, accounting for more deaths than any other cancer of the female reproductive system. A woman's risk of getting this deadly disease during her lifetime is about 1 in 78. Tracy is aware of these statistics as her maternal great-grandmother, aunt, and mother all experienced this cancer that begins in the ovaries.

Her mom recovered from a stage 4 diagnosis and is alive ten years later; the hospital staff refers to her mom as the miracle baby. Her great-grandmother and aunt succumbed to the disease. While Tracy accepts this is a strong family history, she doesn't live in fear that this is her fate. Instead, she uses genetic information to foster a healthy internal and external environment so that tumor growth is unlikely. Her focus is on wellness, not on illness. Tracy credits her mom's recovery in part to a strong mind/body connection and a ceaseless belief that she would get well.

Gabor Maté, MD, who wrote *When the Body Says No,* says that we could prevent and heal many diseases if we fully understood the scientific evidence that shows the mind and body are one. He encourages self-examination, insight, and inspired change. It's empowering to learn we may have more control over our reality and quality of health than we think.

Dr. Maté believes that by acknowledging the mind-body connection, we can address the root causes of illness and achieve real healing. He emphasizes the importance of taking responsibility for our health and making conscious choices that support both our physical and mental health. Maintaining a relationship with a healthcare provider is important, but remember, you are the expert on you!

By understanding the power of our thoughts, we can manifest positive outcomes and attract abundance into our lives. It is important to cultivate a positive mindset and practice mindful awareness to harness this dimension's potential for personal growth and fulfillment. The mind has the ability to influence our emotions, behaviors, and physical health. By tapping into the power of our mind and creating new positive pathways, we can overcome challenges, achieve our goals, and increase our vitality.

I am okay, even when I'm feeling sad, disappointed, or worried
I am learning to trust my body
I am supported by those around me
I am healthy and strong
Thank you
I am grateful to my body for all it does
I am safe in my body
I am aware my sensations are here to guide me
I am love

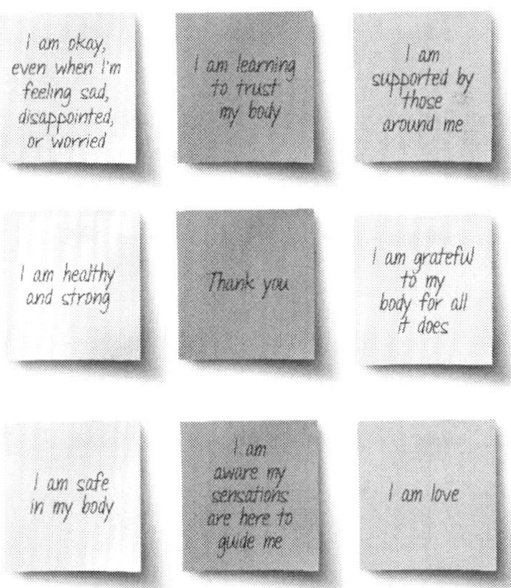

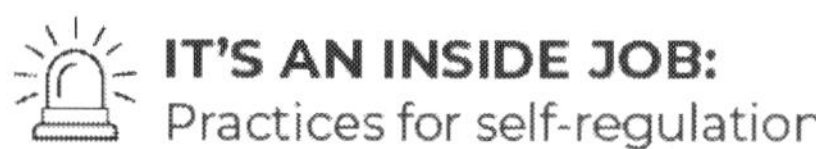

Expanding your understanding of what makes you YOU may be the most significant gift you can give yourself. If 95% of who you are is an unconscious set of behaviors, emotional reactions, unconscious habits, hardwired beliefs, thoughts, and perceptions—who is driving your bus? Be curious; take the wheel! Don't let your subconscious shape your future.

Be a Witness to Your Thoughts

Witnessing your thoughts means being consciously aware of them. Try observing them without judgment or attachment. Remember, you are not your thoughts; they are simply passing through.

Choose Desirable Ones

Once you are aware of your thoughts, you can choose which ones to focus on and give attention to. Remember, repetitive positive thoughts will create new neural pathways that your subconscious mind will draw on to shape your actions. This can help shift your mindset toward creating more positive and productive thinking.

Look for Repetitive Patterns

If you notice the same negative thoughts resurfacing, it may be helpful to examine why they keep coming up. There may be an underlying need that is calling for attention and care. By exploring these patterns, you can begin to address the root causes of your negative thoughts and find ways to fulfill those underlying needs. Seeking guidance from a coach or therapist can help you navigate and understand these patterns more deeply.

Practices for Positive Thinking

Affirmations are positive statements that you repeat to yourself daily, such as "I am capable and deserving of success." By consistently reinforcing these positive beliefs, you can rewire your subconscious mind to believe in your abilities and attract more positivity into your life. Write down positive affirmations on sticky notes and place them around your living space as a visual reminder. Try repeating them aloud throughout the day.

Additionally, you can try visualization techniques where you imagine yourself achieving your goals and feeling the positive emotions associated with them. Create a vision board with images and words that represent your goals and aspirations. By visualizing these affirmations, you are reinforcing their power and bringing them into reality.

Another practice for positive thinking is gratitude. Take a few moments each day to reflect on what you are grateful for and write them down in a gratitude journal. This can help shift your focus towards the positive aspects of your life and cultivate a more optimistic mindset. Additionally, surrounding yourself with positive people and engaging in activities that bring you joy can also contribute to maintaining a positive mindset.

Emotional

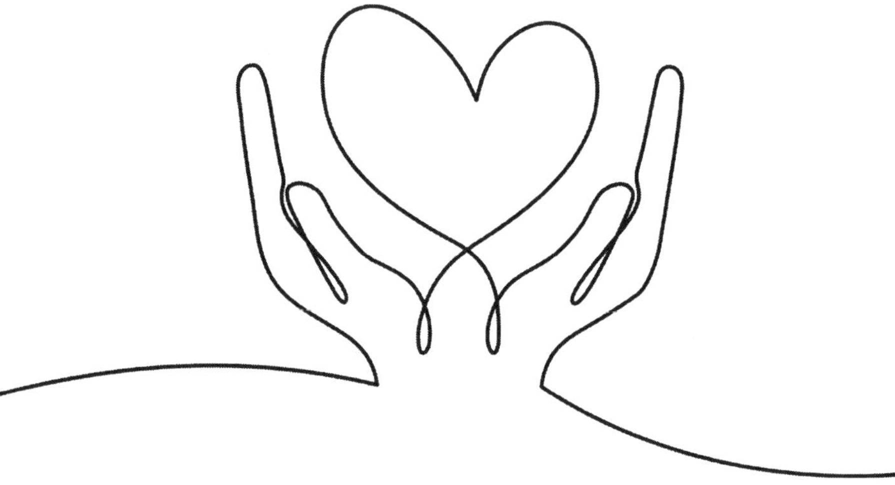

I am in my body
and feel the
sensations that come
up to guide me.

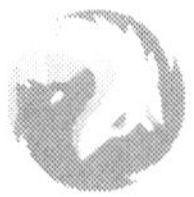

The Tale of Two Wolves

One evening, an elderly Cherokee tells his grandchild about a battle.

"My dear one, the battle between two 'wolves' is inside us all.

One is anger. It embodies envy, jealousy, sorrow, regret, greed, arrogance, self-pity, guilt, resentment, inferiority, lies, false pride, superiority, and ego.

The other is joy. It personifies peace, love, hope, serenity, humility, kindness, benevolence, empathy, truth, compassion, and faith."

The grandchild thought for a moment and then asked the elder: "Which wolf wins?"

The old Cherokee smiled and replied, "If you acknowledge them right, they both win." The story goes on. "You see, if I only listen to the joyful wolf, the angry wolf will hide in the dark, waiting for me to falter so it can pounce and get the attention it craves. The angry wolf will always be fighting the joyful wolf. But if I acknowledge anger, it will be satisfied.

The angry wolf has qualities that I need and that the joyful wolf lacks: tenacity, courage, fearlessness, the strength of will, and resourcefulness. The joyful wolf instead provides compassion, caring, heart, and the ability to value the needs of others over my own.

You see, the two wolves need each other. Feeding only one and starving the other will eventually make both uncontrollable. Caring for both allows them to serve you so you can do something greater and good with your time on earth. Acknowledge them both, and you will quiet their internal struggle for your attention, and when there is no battle inside, you can hear the voices of deeper knowing that will guide you in choosing the right path in every circumstance."

How you treat the opposing forces within you will ultimately determine your level of peace and happiness.

Chapter 4

Emotional Wellness

Writing this book has been an embodied experience for the three of us. We meet each Monday to discuss our progress and, inevitably, spend time sharing experiences, regulation practices, and wisdom gained from our lifelong journeys. As a result, Mondays have become our favorite day of the work week.

We've learned that real connection happens when we let go of our fear of what will happen if we speak our truths. Through this process, we have discovered the power of vulnerability and the strength that comes from being authentic. We have cultivated a deep trust and understanding by creating a safe space for open and honest dialogue.

One week in particular, Helen recounted a childhood experience that was painful for her. While Tracy and Diane felt honored by her trust, Helen felt vulnerable. Recognizing the impact of her past experiences on her present self, Helen shares her process of acknowledging and comforting her inner child.

"Last week, when I shared that childhood experience with you, I felt a profound release from within. Thank you. Being able to do that shows how safe I am with the two of you. But it was a multilayered experience because I've only shared that with two other people.

Later that night, I suddenly felt this sharp feeling throughout my body. It was the victim-like energy of shame and vulnerability that led to a sense of panic. 'What did I do? Why did I share that?' It became a visceral burning sensation. I closed my eyes, took a deep breath, comforted the little kid within, and said, 'I know you are anxious, I know you are afraid, but I got you, I got you. What do you need right now? I'm here.'

Learning to comfort my little kid allows me to give her what she never got when feeling vulnerable. I felt the shame and vulnerability ease when I could meet the discomfort and give myself the love and compassion I needed. We tend to offer tenderness to others freely and don't recognize how liberating it is to give it to ourselves. It was powerful.

Time and again, there is fear of what will happen when we allow ourselves to be vulnerable, but with this process, it is possible to comfort and heal old wounds. That was releasing stuck energy. That was energy in motion."

Searching for solutions to what keeps us from living a life of ease is not found out there somewhere; the answers are inside us. By learning to let our emotions lead us instead of resisting them or identifying with them, we can bring simplicity to what initially seems to be our most complex dimension. Observing, feeling, and letting the emotional energy pass through us without resistance are all part of this practice. We hope sharing our experiences sparks something in YOU that leads to greater self-awareness, healing, and more room for joy. Helen's ability to be present in her body when emotions arise allows her to be with her emotional discomfort instead of reaching for a crutch to quell what is burning within, retreating, or acting out in a manner that isn't productive. You might surmise that she's been practicing for some time, and she has. How beautiful and healing it is to bring love and compassion to places of pain. We'll talk more about Helen's effective practices, but first, let's cover some basics.

> **Emotional wellness is understanding ourselves and embracing all of life's challenges. It is acknowledging, accepting, befriending, and sharing feelings of anger, fear, sadness, distress, hope, love, joy, and happiness in a productive manner.**

There is no health without emotional health. Emotional health is foundational. With a curious lens, we can understand why we are triggered. Why are we stuck? Why do we repeat patterns in life and relationships? Why do we feel sad? The more awareness we have about ourselves, the more effectively we can navigate life.

Before we talk about what emotions are, let's talk about what they are not— feelings. While they are often used interchangeably, they have distinct differences. Emotions are instinctive; they are subconscious reactions to physical experiences. Information from our environment gets processed through the nervous system and triggers an emotion.

On the other hand, feelings are conscious reactions to these emotions expressed in thoughts. As emotions happen in the body, feelings occur in the mind. They are the mind's interpretation of the body's state. Individual beliefs, experiences, and thoughts all impact feelings, which can vary from person to person. Additionally, while emotions are often fleeting and temporary, feelings can be more enduring and have a longer-lasting impact on our overall well-being.

The mind narrates what the body already knows.

Since emotions happen first, let's dig deeper before discussing our feelings. Emotions = (E)energy in (Motion)

When we think about emotions, we think about movement since they are continuously working to regulate our cells to adapt to threats, opportunities, and everything in between. According to Dr. Jill Bolte Taylor, a Harvard-trained and published neuroscientist, 90 seconds is all it takes for an emotion to move through the body and dissipate. "When a person reacts to something in their environment, there's a 90-second chemical process that happens in the body; any remaining emotional response is just the person choosing to stay in that emotional loop," she explains.

In a little more than a minute, an emotion moves through the body to where we subconsciously attach to or release it. But, just as we discovered in the intellectual chapter, the most empowering realization is that with conscious awareness, we have the power to choose how we respond. This conscious choice is the difference between something happening to us or for us.

The ability to choose doesn't mean we are happy all the time. Instead, we continue to experience all our emotions in response to our environment and bring awareness to them without judgment. This self-awareness empowers us to make conscious choices about how we want to respond instead of reacting automatically without pausing for consideration.

When we pause and reflect on our feelings, we can work to better understand ourselves and the reasons behind our reactions. This self-reflection allows us to break free from automatic, unconscious responses and practice accepting and befriending our emotions while cultivating understanding through a more compassionate lens. This process enables us to develop greater control over our lives and foster personal growth and development.

Emotions serve as valuable indicators of our inner world and can guide us toward understanding our needs and desires. We can cultivate deeper self-awareness and personal growth by embracing our emotions and allowing them to guide us. What remains true is that emotions are our friends.

Emotions carry essential messages and wisdom about our needs, fears, and truths.

Wisdom of joy: Joy is the emotion of delight; there is a lightness in the body when experiencing something positive.

Wisdom of anger: Anger is the body trying to protect us! It says, "My needs are valid, I am asking for respect, and my voice counts. I matter."

Wisdom of sadness: Sadness lets us know we are experiencing hurt or grief over something meaningful.

Wisdom of happiness: Happiness is a sense of contentment; the body conveys a message of spaciousness and well-being.

Wisdom of fear: Fear is a warning signal. It is the body's way of asking us to pay attention.

Wisdom of shame: Shame is linked to feelings of imperfection, self-loathing, or inadequacy. It is the body's way of telling us it is time to practice self-love.

Instead of seeing emotions as good or bad, we can start to see them as energy designed to move through our bodies, providing clues for how to respond to life. In addition, it's necessary to have opposing emotions to enjoy a rich and full life experience; it would be hard to revel in something joyous if you never knew sorrow. By learning to turn toward our emotions and feelings instead of away from them, we can create a new world for ourselves with greater happiness and ease. Learning to recognize and lean into her sensations was a turning point in Tracy's life:

"Suffering from chronic Lyme Disease and desperate for answers to what was happening in my body, I started Quantum Biofeedback therapy for some alternative insight. Through electrical sensors attached to the ankles, wrists, and head, a medical software program scans the body, like a computer virus scan, and monitors involuntary functions to help relay what is happening on a cellular level. I would marvel at the results and how accurately the findings matched my symptoms. The reports were fascinating, except I couldn't fathom the possibility of a software program reading my emotions; it seemed highly implausible. Not to mention, the results didn't jive. Time and time again, anger appeared as the number-one emotion I was experiencing. What?!

Fear? Yes.
Limited belief in oneself? Yup.
Unsure of my place in the world? Okay, yes.
ANGER? I am the least angry person I know.

I ignored all this emotional nonsense and, over time, managed to get well. The Lyme and accompanying pathogens resurfaced with a vengeance a few years later, and by this time, I was aware of its purpose: to enlighten me. Along with countless other practitioners, I revisited my friendly biofeedback specialist, and wouldn't you know, anger still appeared in the number-one spot like a dark horse. This time, I was ready to go there. Not only was I entirely unaware of the anger I was harboring, but I also began to understand that I didn't feel, nor could I identify, many of the emotions that flowed through me daily. I was stuck; I believe this eventually manifested into disease.

It was here that I understood the need to connect with my body and started my true healing journey."

As a protective mechanism, the body can bury intense emotions. Anger is often used to conceal more complex emotions such as sadness, fear, or grief. The unresolved trauma from Tracy's childhood contributed to turmoil in her adult life, finally manifesting as disease. Only by seeing and acknowledging these aspects of ourselves can they be altered or healed.

I am.

One of the most common mistakes we make is identifying with our feelings. Feelings are something we experience; we are not our feelings. Learning to separate our identity from our feelings is critical to emotional well-being. Saying "I am sad" builds an identity around sadness, whereas "I feel sad" describes what we are experiencing and suggests its impermanence. This perspective allows us to approach our emotions with curiosity and compassion rather than judgment or attachment.

"Feelings are something you have, not something you are."
—Shannon L. Alder

When using "I am," make sure it's positive. I am thankful. I am capable. I am worthy. Our bodies are highly attuned to our thoughts and beliefs, constantly picking up on the messages we send ourselves. Positive "I am" statements can lead to a more optimistic outlook, attracting more positive experiences and opportunities. Let's not forget that the words we choose to define ourselves have a profound effect on our mental health.

We have found that many of us were conditioned in childhood to suppress or ignore naturally occurring feelings, but as we learned in the Tale of Two Wolves, feelings will fight to be expressed one way or another. The elder Cherokee states that we must recognize and welcome ALL feelings to quiet the battle inside. We can create a healthier and more balanced emotional landscape by embracing the idea that all feelings are valid and should be acknowledged and accepted.

Consequences of suppressed feelings may include:

— Anxiousness

— Agitation

— Fear

— Depression

— Anger

— Addiction

— Low self-esteem and low self-worth

— Unhealthy relationships

— Chronic pain

— Disease

When we ignore our feelings, we resist them instead of allowing them to flow. That resistance energy gets trapped in our body and, like clutter, can build up over time. As the elder Cherokee so aptly describes, our feelings will hide in the dark, waiting for us to falter so they can pounce and get the attention they crave. Children often cannot process strong emotions because they are overwhelmed by their experiences or worried the feelings will last forever. They don't yet have the language to convey this or the ability to self-regulate. Suppressed emotions may continue to impact us, manifesting as physical symptoms or unhealthy coping mechanisms.

Stay curious. Your patterns are trying to tell you something.

As our conscious attention grows, we may notice patterns. Repeatedly finding ourselves in the same undesirable situation might mean we are stuck. Being caught in an unwanted cycle can be frustrating and disheartening, but it is essential to remember that we have the power to heal and grow. Be curious about recurring thoughts and behaviors. Knowing our "whys" is our greatest source of wisdom. By acknowledging and addressing our repetitive patterns, we can begin the process of healing them.

The brain uses patterns to keep us safe because they allow us to predict the future. However, we are unable to reconcile what we don't know. Once we spot the pattern, we can step back and view it through a wider lens. Asking ourselves questions with the same compassion we would for a close friend or a young child helps us uncover what shapes these behaviors:

What emotions or fears are driving these patterns?
Are there underlying beliefs or thoughts that are contributing to them?
What fundamental needs are not being met?

Chances are this coping mechanism protected you at one point, but how we learned to survive in the past may not serve us in the present. By understanding the root causes of our patterns, we can bring compassion to those places and consciously adopt new ways of being that align with our current needs and goals. What are you tethered to that needs to be healed?

Self-awareness and empathy are the roots of EQ.

Emotional Intelligence first appeared in the early 1960s but gained popularity with the book by psychologist Daniel Goleman, Ph.D., *Emotional Intelligence: Why It Can Matter More Than IQ.* Emotional intelligence (emotional quotient or EQ) can help us connect with our feelings and build stronger relationships. Engaging our EQ means using our emotions to make constructive decisions about our behaviors. For example, we increase our tolerance by staying present in uncomfortable places without letting them override our thoughts and self-control.

Diane tells an amusing story about when she told her son to stop breathing at the top of a Ferris wheel. What does that have to do with EQ? Let's back up a little and let her explain:

"When I was a pre-teen, I was excited the day I had the opportunity to ride an amusement park ride with my older brothers. Much to the delight of my brothers, when the ride stopped, our car kept spinning. It felt like we were spinning out of control for hours. I kept twisting in my seat to see what was happening; I was terrified and worried something awful would happen. I'm sure it was only seconds and just one or two extra rotations; we were fine when the car finally stopped. My brothers were thrilled. While I should have allowed myself to cry, scream, or ask for a hug, I didn't do anything to release my terror. Instead, I have carried that energy with me all these years, and I'm still not fond of amusement park rides.

All three of my kids love rides. For them, the faster, the higher, the more twists, the better. So, when they were little, I took them to New York City for Mother's Day to ride the indoor Ferris wheel at their favorite toy store. Since the Ferris wheel had an enclosed bucket seat instead of a single-line, exposed carriage, I thought I could handle it—famous last words. I was okay until we stopped at the very top. My son thought this was great; he saw the whole store and started moving in his seat, making the bucket sway. I'm sure I subconsciously heard my brother's excited laughter, which triggered panic. Through gritted teeth, I told my son in my best mom's voice, "Do not move, do not look around, don't even BREATHE."

Yup, Mom of the Year, I was not. There was no self-awareness, self-regulation, or EQ; I let the situation override my self-control. So, instead of giving them this fantastic and fun experience, I gave my kids a glimpse of their mom at her most vulnerable. Fortunately, it's a story they all still laugh about, sometimes laughing uncontrollably until they can hardly breathe.

I appreciate that the 'incident' did not alter our relationship, create fear, or affect their love for adventure. Instead, their grace and compassion (com-

bined with laughter) allowed me to accept my humanity. It was, however, a wake-up call for me to better understand myself and develop tools for self-regulation, to learn that discomfort does not necessarily mean danger."

Each of our three stories relates to an unresolved wound we experienced in childhood that continues to affect us in the present. We know that trauma can happen because of an abusive situation, a natural disaster, a crime, a war, or life-altering events that are easy to recognize. But it's much broader than that; our bodies retain memories of any experience that overwhelmed us at the time and was left unresolved, and those imprinted recollections continue to impact us today.

A seemingly benign wound in childhood can impact our ability to cope, cause feelings of helplessness, affect our ability to experience a full range of emotions, and keep us from living to our fullest potential as adults. While a spinning amusement park ride doesn't merit a life-changing event, it manifests in Diane's need to control her environment and a desire to stay in a safe zone regarding fun and adventure.

Moreover, it is a very personalized emotion. Diane's story also serves as an excellent illustration of how experiences present differently for different people; her brothers enjoyed the same event that traumatized her. How often have you heard a relative tell a story about a family event you experienced together that leaves you wondering if you were in the same place? Trauma is not the event itself but rather our response to the event.

Due to the subjective nature of trauma, there is no foolproof method of objectively assessing the severity of its potential consequences. Physical abuse, rejection, humiliation, racism, harassment, and misuse of power are all examples of harmful behaviors that can affect us at any age. For a child, though, trauma can also be defined by what didn't happen and should have, specifically failure to meet a child's foundational needs. Even loving parents can unintentionally raise a child who feels broken and incomplete as an adult. It took Tracy years to discover what specific unmet needs were driving her dis-ease; filling those needs by reparenting herself became crucial to her healing journey.

Because the body is designed to protect us, the brain can suppress these experiences; this is often protective for us in the short term. However, over time, trapped emotions can lead to dysregulation. The body remembers. And because the unprocessed energy is stored at the cellular level, the body may re-experience the trauma anytime a trigger evokes the related emotion.

We can see our triggers as flashing lights reminding us of what needs to be healed. It is common to think, "Other people's struggles and traumas are worse than mine." While that may be true, it doesn't take away from our wounds or make them any less real. What we carry can still be heavy; the body remembers what the mind allows us to hide away. Until we normalize the idea that we are all struggling with something nobody knows about, we will continue to bring wounded energy to the greater collective. If we each focus on identifying and healing our emotional scars, imagine the impact on our futures and the world!

> *"Trauma is not what happens to us, but what we hold inside in the absence of an empathetic witness."* —Peter A. Levine

Our three stories demonstrate that each of us has experienced trauma of various kinds and intensities. Helen keeps making connections and letting go of trauma energy on her own and with the help of a somatic experienced therapist. Tracy continues to research and carry out similar work, and Diane uses emotional intelligence to make good decisions about how to act in response to her past trauma. In our unique ways, we have found that the more we empty the body of unresolved issues, the more space there is for us to cultivate love and joy.

Suppressed emotions can prevent us from living our best lives. We must work to uncover what we are harboring and how it affects us, or we risk continually returning to our negative patterns and comfort zones. It is essential to acknowledge that healing is a journey that takes time. By being patient with ourselves and practicing self-compassion, we can create a safe space for our emotions to surface and be released.

As Helen describes, compassion is necessary to lighten our load. Imagine the space created in the body when a single molecule of love interacts with a single molecule of pain. We unlock the door to healing when we love and care for ourselves like we would a small child. By being aware of and accepting our feelings, we can give the body permission to release them and make room for the future we want to create. This allows us to move forward with a clearer mind and a lighter heart.

So, where do I begin?

You already have. The first step is always awareness. Are you stuck? What do you fear? What might need tending to? What brings you joy? Begin to listen to your thoughts and watch your behaviors as a witness. Remember, there is nothing wrong with you! You make perfect sense. Honor your journey. In an environment of safety and support, curiosity and compassion can take you where you need to go.

IT'S AN INSIDE JOB:
Practices for self-regulation

Emotion = energy in motion. Moving our emotions is crucial to managing them effectively. However, when we attach to them, or they become overwhelming, our behaviors and relationships can be negatively impacted. We can use tools like the following exercises to help keep things in motion.

Turn Up the Volume!

Our friend Jill Teas is the co-founder and conductor of an adult rock choir in Denver, CO. Voices Rock aims to build a sense of belonging and connection through music. The participants report increased happiness and an overall higher sense of well-being during their sessions. Singing stimulates blood and oxygen flow to your brain, improving cognitive function and enhancing mood. Additionally, singing releases endorphins, or natural feel-good chemicals, that can reduce stress and anxiety.

Try belting out an upbeat tune the next time you find yourself in an emotional rut. Singing can be a simple yet effective way to improve your emotional well-being. It doesn't matter how you sound; sing! Think of it as a natural anti-depressant.

Unleash Your Inner Lion

Lion's Breath is a breathing technique that helps to release stress and tension from the body and mind. Sit in a comfortable and stable position.

1. With your eyes open, inhale deeply through your nose.

2. Open your mouth and stick your tongue out.

3. Exhale, making a long "ha" sound.

Repeat this exercise a few times. Then, take a moment to notice any changes or sensations that arise; notice if there is space created in the body. Letting go of any self-judgment will enable you to try this exercise with child-like ease.

Shake It Off

According to Dr. Peter Levine, in his book Waking the Tiger, animals use shaking to release trauma energy from their bodies. The stress cycle has a beginning, middle, and end. We often cannot complete the process in stressful situations, and energy remains in the body. Research suggests we can release stress and complete the cycle by shaking the body.

Try this: Take a deep, cleansing breath and notice how you feel in your body. Now, vigorously shake your arms, legs, feet, and hips. Don't be afraid to get a little goofy. Channel your inner pop star and "Shake it Off!" Notice if you feel differently before and after.

> Recently, Tracy used the "Shake it off" technique to release trauma energy at an unimaginable event. At a banquet celebrating one of her sisters, Tracy's father choked at dinner and went into respiratory arrest, shocking her and her family. Tracy's mom and siblings asked her to accompany her dad in an ambulance to the hospital as medics worked to save his life. As she was given instructions for her role in the triage unit, Tracy's arms and legs began to go numb. Recognizing the signs of excess adrenaline, she knew what to do. She could discharge the energy and regain control of her body by jumping up and down and vigorously shaking her arms and legs. Tragically, her father lost his life in the triage unit. But, because of this practice, Tracy was able to restore her composure and be fully present when he passed.

Social

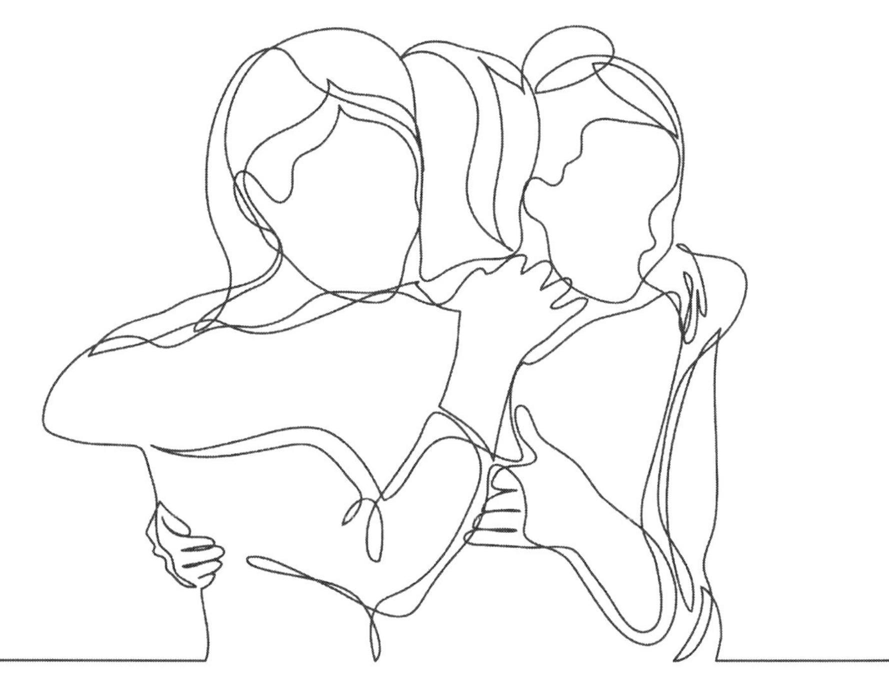

I am connected
to myself and those
around me.

"Encourage, lift, and strengthen one another.
For the positive energy spread to one will be felt by us all.
For we are connected, one and all."

—Deborah Day

Chapter 5

Social Wellness

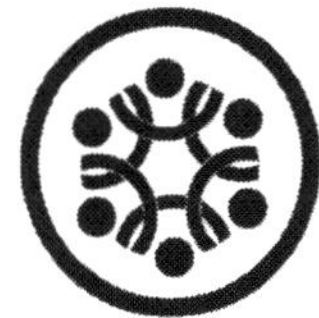

What brings the three of us together to write this book is a collective belief in the wisdom of our experiences. We hope the desire to share our stories sparks something in you, dear friend. Sharing pain and joy unites us; the human experience is our bond.

Each of us has a unique background—our circumstances, upbringing, and life experiences vary greatly. We have discovered that building meaningful relationships with people whose core values complement our own while having different insights, proficiencies, and life experiences enables us to create a more balanced and colorful life experience.

Close friends don't just increase our pleasure; they can help us manage stress. Conversing with a trusted friend is a great way to bring a sense of safety and calm to our nervous systems. It turns out this practice has a name: co-regulation. According to Dr. Leaf, Ph.D., as we co-regulate with someone, mirror neurons in the brain are activated, enabling the person in the deregulated state to literally "mirror" calmness. Studies show people with meaningful relationships live longer and have more joy, hope, and happiness. It's important to note that the quality of relationships matters more than the quantity. It's not about having a large group of friends but rather having meaningful relationships that provide emotional support and a sense of connection.

Social wellness is establishing and nurturing positive relationships with self, family, friends, and co-workers while maintaining healthy boundaries. It is realizing that every relationship we have is directly impacted by how we feel about ourselves.

Humans are hard-wired to connect, but the need alone isn't enough. Many of us find ourselves increasingly disconnected and feeling alone. Authentic connections require vulnerability and openness. By being honest about our own struggles and needs, we create a foundation for genuine relationships that can provide the emotional support and sense of connection necessary for social wellness.

"Being able to feel safe with other people is probably the single most important aspect of mental health; safe connections are fundamental to meaningful and satisfying lives." —Bessel A. van der Kolk

To maintain authentic connections with others, we must continuously work on self-awareness and self-reflection. This involves regularly checking in with ourselves to understand our own emotions, needs, and boundaries. When we find ourselves repeating unhealthy relationship patterns, it may be time to bring awareness to subconscious needs from our past that remain unmet.

Are you my mother?

Consider that our relationships begin the moment we are born, and our earliest experiences reflect how we navigate the world. We learn how to interact with others and develop ways to express ourselves through our most primitive bonds. Our earliest memories remind us of how our caregivers conditioned us to communicate our needs and respond to the world around us.

For most of us, our first gift of nourishment is our mother's milk. At birth, sustenance, safety, and love are our most primal necessities; they drive our need for bonding. With the understanding that we experience life in the nervous system, this is where we first sense how our caregivers are meeting our needs.

Attachment, or the attachment bond, a fundamental concept in psychology and child development, is the emotional connection we form as infants with our primary caregivers. According to British psychiatrist John Bowlby and American psychologist Mary Ainsworth, the bonding quality we experience during this first relationship often determines how well we relate to other people and respond to intimacy throughout life.

With a sense of curious awareness and compassion, we can search for connections between our earliest bonds with our caregivers and our relationship patterns as adults. According to holistic psychologist Dr. Nicole LePera, learning which early attachment style resonates most with you can help make these connections. Dr. LePera's work aligns with a comprehensive approach to mental health, emphasizing the interconnectedness of mind, body, and spirit.

It's important to note that attachment styles are not static and can change with time and personal growth. As we gain self-awareness and engage in healing practices, we have the potential to shift our attachment style towards a more secure and healthy pattern. This transformation can lead to more fulfilling and satisfying relationships in adulthood. Attachment styles are commonly categorized into several types, including:

Secure. A securely attached infant may get upset for a brief period after the caregiver leaves but will recover quickly. When the caregiver returns, the child is open and receptive to the reunion. The caregiver appears to have provided a safe and stable environment.
Anxious-resistant. The infant may be so stressed and distressed by the caregiver's absence that they remain upset the entire time the caregiver is gone. When they return, the child isn't comforted easily— this type of bond results from a mix-attunement between the child's needs and the caregiver's attention.
Avoidant. Children in this category show almost no stress response when the mother leaves and virtually no reaction when the caregiver returns. Typically, this response is the product of a disconnected parent figure who leaves the child to navigate independently. The child doesn't go to the parent figure for help with their emotional state because the parent figure doesn't provide that support.
Disorganized-disoriented. These children show no predictable pattern of response. Sometimes, they are completely distressed, and sometimes, they show no reaction at all. This rarest attachment style is typically associated with childhood trauma. The child's world is so unpredictable that their body doesn't know how to react or find safety.

A child feels safer and more confident in the world the closer and more secure their relationship is with their immediate parental figures. According to numerous studies, those who form secure attachments as babies are likelier to do so as adults. Dr. LePera also asserts a connection between social anxiety and a child's inability to develop secure attachments.

Can you identify with an attachment bond and connect it to how you relate to others in the present? Tracy acknowledges that she had an attachment wound. Growing up in a large family, she believes she missed the care and support she needed during critical periods of her childhood. Through the lens of her younger self, Tracy experienced feelings of fear and abandonment as she navigated seemingly alone.

Although she doesn't believe this was her parents' intention, Tracy believed being herself was an affliction. An unmet need for safety, recognition, and emotional support became a roadblock that impacted how she saw and handled herself and her relationships as an adult. If you resonate with this example or feel like being "you" is a burden to others, it isn't reality. More than likely, it is how you perceive reality based on childhood experiences. Tracy's beliefs were deeply rooted in her subconscious and appeared as unhealthy patterns. These strategies will repeat until we are ready to confront and heal the underlying wounds from our past.

After years of self-sabotage, Tracy learned to feel her emotions and ask into her pain, "What deep need is behind my beliefs and behaviors?" Along with awareness, acceptance, and self-love, the work for her became letting go of the idea that she didn't have a choice to move forward. Healing doesn't tickle, but finding a way to care for our unmet needs allows us to show up as our true selves. Authenticity unlocks the door to the connection we're longing for.

Even if you didn't have secure attachment bonds growing up, you may still be able to extend grace to your parents. Imagine giving *them* everything they needed for a life of safety and fulfillment; how might they have cared for you differently? How might *they* be different? Giving them compassion and grace can lighten your load and help heal generational wounds.

If you're willing to be curious about what attachment style you see yourself in, remember there is absolutely nothing wrong with you. You make perfect sense. The most crucial relationship for wellness and ease is our relationship with ourselves; building that relationship begins from a place of compassion.

Your most important relationship is YOU!

Every other relationship you have is influenced by how you feel about yourself. How you love yourself is how you teach others to love you. When someone doesn't respect you, it's not that they don't see your value; in fact, they probably do. They know YOU don't value yourself, so you let them treat you that way, too.

When we talk about developing a relationship with ourselves, it means developing an understanding of ourselves at all ages—each stage of our development is a part of who we are. We are the sum of our experiences. Many trace the concept of our inner child to psychiatrist Carl Jung, who described a child archetype in his work. He linked this internal child to past experiences and memories of innocence, playfulness, creativity, and hope for the future. Other experts describe this inner child concept as an expression of not just our child self but our experiences at all stages of life.

When childhood experiences negatively affect us, our inner child may continue to carry these wounds until we address them in our body in the present. When we find our inner child in a place of suffering, we can help them heal, bringing lightness to our being. At the same time, our inner child at different stages and times can also lend *us* strength. For example, regaining youthful feelings of wonder, optimism, and simple joy in life can help bolster confidence and well-being. Isn't that what friends are for?

> *"Your inner child needs a hero, and that hero is the powerful person that stands before you in the mirror."* —Danny Brave

One of our most significant realizations is that the brain cannot distinguish who is speaking. This means the same neural pathways are activated whether we listen to our thoughts or someone else's voice. As a result, we can be our own best friend or greatest adversary. This discovery highlights the power of self-talk and the importance of being kind to ourselves. Being our worst critic and engaging in negative self-talk can harm our mental health and well-being.

On the other hand, when we treat ourselves with the same compassion and understanding we would offer to a friend, we can build a strong sense of self-worth and self-confidence, favorably impacting our relationships with others. Tracy uses this self-guided visualization to meet her younger self, where she gives her the love and compassion she longed for and deserves:

"I close my eyes and step into an elevator, traveling to a level deep inside myself. I am set to arrive at a magical garden that is beyond comparison. As the doors open, I see a little girl on a bench waiting patiently for me. She IS me, in fact, at an earlier age. We sit together, and I feel her worry as I gaze into her eyes. I begin to tell her everything she needs to hear. I tell her she is safe and will never be alone; I will always be right here. I put her hand in mine, press it against my heart, and say, 'There is nothing to worry about, Sweetheart. Nothing can happen that you and I cannot handle together.' I ask her to let go, be free, and dance. And for a moment, I embrace her with all my love and then send her on her way. As I sit among the flowering trees, I watch her run, spin, and dance away—carefree. I love her; she is a part of who I am, and I am releasing her voice of worry."

Notice how gentle and reassuring she is. By allowing herself to feel the fear in the eyes of her younger self, Tracy can heal her with her love and support. In effect, she is reparenting herself. Take a breath, go inside, and notice where you are.

If befriending yourself at certain ages feels uncomfortable, give yourself grace and know it's okay. You may want to consider exploring these emotions with a trained practitioner. If your response is one of curiosity, make Tracy's exercise your own and explore the opportunity to reparent yourself.

I'm feeling alone in a sea of people.

Even for some of us with solid attachment bonds, the isolation we experienced during the pandemic negatively impacted our mental health. Some became fearful and stuck in a state of fight-or-flight because the pandemic disrupted our lives in ways we had never imagined before. On the other hand, some found solace in this same isolation. It helped us grow closer to the people in our inner circles and allowed us to establish new boundaries in our lives. To create practices that help us return to a sense of safety and connection, it can be helpful to remember that our bodies are designed to handle stress, anxiety, grief, and worry during trying times.

We can't think about social wellness and the pandemic without talking about loneliness. It's important to understand that sometimes loneliness is hard to identify because it is a subjective experience. It occurs when our desired social relationships do not resemble our actual relationships.

Try not to confuse solitude with loneliness or isolation. Solitude is a state of being where we are alone but not lonely. It can be an opportunity to recharge and reflect on our thoughts and emotions. Solitude is a healthy and necessary part of self-care. Loneliness is a state of mind. It's the feeling of isolation and disconnection from others, even in a crowded room. Loneliness is often involuntary and can lead to negative emotions and depression. Studies show that loneliness is rising; some say it has steadily increased since the 1970s. Evidence shows that individuals who feel lonely or spend time in isolation are more likely to suffer from mental and physical health issues. Are we losing our ability to connect?

Social anxiety is a type of *dis*-ease that can lead to loneliness and isolation. A common misconception about individuals with social anxiety is that they are antisocial. In reality, many with this mental health condition are very anxious about being around others and find social interactions exhausting. According to the Mayo Clinic, social anxiety is more than everyday nervousness; it includes fear, anxiety, and avoidance that interferes with relationships, daily routines, work, school, or other activities.

As we discussed in the first chapter, our bodies need to be in the right physical state to be actively social. When we are in an activated state, our ability to use our social system suffers. We understand genuine connection necessitates honesty and trust, but our past experiences in childhood can make us feel fearful and unsafe.

Mark, the father of Diane's children, died of ALS at just 43 years old; they had previously divorced due in part to Mark's alcoholism. Their youngest child, Nick, was just 4 when they divorced and only 13 at the time of Mark's death. This horrible disease wreaked havoc on Mark's body and then on her children's mental health for years to come. While each child has had their own path, anxiety and fear of loss became a common thread. The attachment bond between Mark and Nick was strong. When Mark was fully present, he was a wonderful dad who greatly impacted Nick as a child; he helped shape Nick into the empathetic, brave, and self-confident person he is today.

Until recently, Nick was not ready to face his grief or childhood trauma. Then, at 31 years old, he boldly decided to leave a lucrative yet toxic career and move to Vietnam, where he could work on creating a life in line with his values while experiencing more of the world.

Through the years, Diane and Nick developed a strong bond with good, honest verbal communication. They can be very vulnerable with each other, and Nick now fully appreciates that asking for help is a sign of strength. However, now that he is a world away, sometimes Diane wonders if there are still many unspoken words in their text messages. She imagines they might read like this:

Diane: Hi, honey. How are you?

Nick: Hi, Mom. Sorry it took so long to respond, I've been ~~anxious and lonely, taking long walks to clear my head, gave up drinking, tried journaling but don't know what to write, and I'm sleeping in a lot~~ really busy.

Diane: So nice to hear from you! I really miss you. The house is too quiet – are you settled in now?

Nick: I ~~am overwhelmed, isolating, completely drained, and second-guessing this decision, Vietnam is not what I expected~~, found a cafe that I like a lot and met some nice people.

Diane: That's great! How is the job?

Nick: I think ~~I had a panic attack, did a lot of deep breathing, finally got my composure, I definitely had a migraine, I'm not sure I fit in, I'm in over my head~~, it's going to work out well.

Diane: Great. Can we FaceTime tomorrow? I really miss seeing you. ~~I'm worried about you~~. Love you lots, xo

Nick: Sure, say hi to everyone, love you too xo

Loneliness can sometimes feel shameful. When we feel shame, we direct our focus inward and can only see ourselves through the lens that something is wrong with us. Sadly, it's easy to understand why lonely people may think they are unlovable or undesirable; these are false conclusions created in the mind.

What if it's possible to relieve this suffering?

Russell Kennedy, MD, a neuroscientist and the author of *Anxiety Rx*, claims that all anxiety is separation anxiety or an intense fear of being cut off from one's SELF. He asserts that people with anxiety once stopped believing in love because they thought it wasn't safe; this typically occurs during childhood.

Any situation that exceeds a child's capacity to cope and that is not resolved leads to a dysregulated state; for instance, being bullied, the death or divorce of a parent, a caregiver's ongoing neglect, or physical or mental abuse. Any extreme fear in a child's eyes can overwhelm the body and disrupt the system.

Just as Helen described in her story with the four bricks, the child self-splits or separates as a means of self-preservation. According to Dr. Kennedy, for the child inside us to return to a place of safety and love, the child must know that our adult selves won't reject or abandon us. Tracy's elevator exercise is an example of how we might accomplish this. As we regain the trust in the love that our present-day self gives to our younger self, we resolve the split or separation within us—this is what inner healing looks like.

We know that loneliness and social isolation can factor in early mortality. This fact makes repairing that split in ourselves imperative for our health and well-being. Healing ourselves and finding ways to hold space for others to do the same can have a transformative impact on our overall wellness and, dare we say, a ripple effect on the world around us. As we continue to bring awareness to our social health, we cannot underestimate the power of the company we keep.

Surround yourself with friends who motivate and inspire, encouraging your personal growth.

We know it's cliche, but what we surround ourselves with, we become. As creators of our journeys, we want to surround ourselves with people who reflect the vibration of who we want to be. Tracy's friend Nicole is one of those people. Even our seemingly insignificant interactions with others can hugely affect us. Without our knowledge, our nervous systems become interconnected. Our brains contain "mirror" neurons, which reflect what those around us are going through; this allows us to feel empathy. Some consider mirror neurons one of the most important discoveries in the last decade of neuroscience.

The discovery of mirror neurons has had significant implications for our understanding of social cognition, empathy, imitation, and understanding the actions and intentions of others. These neurons play a role in bridging the gap between our actions and the actions of those around us, enabling us to understand and connect with others on a social and emotional level. While mirror neurons' exact functions and implications continue to be an area of research and exploration, they are considered an important component of our social and cognitive processing.

Suitably, we are more likely to feel optimistic around high vibrational people. We do not imply that we should avoid people just because they're unhappy. On the contrary, just as we would want them to support us during trying times, we may offer support to a friend experiencing emotional difficulty. However, issues arise when someone is constantly negative, and we begin to take that on. Therefore, we must listen closely to the signals our body sends us. The body knows.

Our friend Nicole trained for months to participate in an endurance event in Canada. She flew from her home in Boston to Vancouver only to find her luggage did not make it and may not arrive in time for her event. Instead of becoming the victim of this unfortunate circumstance, Nicole took control of her state of mind and refused to let it ruin her experience. The following is their text exchange after Tracy checked in for an update:

Tracy: I'm so sorry about your luggage situation; how are you?

Nicole: I *chose* not to get angry at the baggage claim clerk, who was not responsible for my bag not arriving.

I *chose* to be positive and not add to the angry drama being spewed by a fellow traveler who was irate about his lost bag and complained about anything and everything wrong with the Vancouver airport.

I chose to get to sleep as soon as possible last night instead of tossing and turning about my bag—the most pressing thing at that moment was getting sleep.

I chose to reach out to (event) staff and participants with my dilemma and got offers immediately to help.

I chose to let myself have a really good cry—something I haven't done for a long, long time. It was freeing and cathartic, and it is over—I had that moment quietly, alone in my hotel room.

I chose to get on the next bus I could to Whistler and will deal with the bag later tonight as best I can.

I will *choose* to enjoy this day and all it has to offer with my sister. I am healthy, and that's a lot to be grateful for.

I will continue to make good choices and let go of everything out of my control.

Tracy: <3 This is beautiful; you brought me to tears. Talk about an inspiring frame of mind! You've already gotten a medal.

What a fantastic response. Our ability to choose is our superpower! We are grateful to have Nicole in our friend group and to have you here, too. No matter what challenges come our way, we can always choose to approach them with a growth mindset and gratitude. Nicole's example serves as a constant reminder to appreciate the things we have and let go of what we cannot change. It's amazing how a simple shift in mindset can bring so much inspiration.

Regardless of how you reacted to the pandemic or how your mindset shifted as you maneuvered the uncharted waters, what is abundantly clear is that social wellness matters. Remember that loneliness is a state of mind; our perceptions may not be reality. If you find yourself persistently lonely, work toward finding ways to increase your connections. The loving-kindness meditation at the end of the Spiritual chapter is an excellent exercise for cultivating self-love. Reaching out to a licensed practitioner may help you break the negative cycle that created your current state of mind.

Imagine if we approached everyone like they were fighting a battle we know nothing about.

How different would the world be if we approached everyone as if they were struggling inside? Interacting with others as if they were fighting a battle we know nothing about is rooted in empathy, compassion, and understanding. This mindset encourages us to be kind, patient, and supportive, recognizing that everyone has burdens and struggles.

While this perspective encourages kindness, it does not suggest that we ignore harmful behaviors or actions. Instead, it focuses on giving others grace rather than judging their experiences. We can foster a sense of unity by recognizing our shared complexities and humanity. This is an invitation to approach all interactions with open-mindedness and empathy.

A small act of goodwill or a kind word can significantly impact someone's life. Together, we can create a better world.

If you or someone you know has thoughts of death or is considering suicide, please get in touch with 988 Suicide & Crisis Lifeline by dialing 988 or by going to their website at 988lifeline.org.

Reach out. Your life matters.

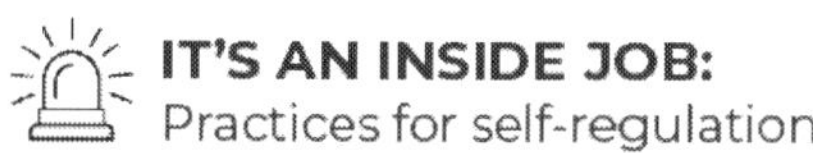

It's common to face recurring challenges in relationships, and it can be frustrating when you're unsure of the underlying reasons. Understanding the root causes of these struggles can help you navigate and improve your connection. Relationship patterns in adulthood can result from the way we bonded in early childhood. There are four styles of attachment that we may develop, and they can influence how we approach and navigate relationships throughout our lives.

Although you may not completely identify with one style, being curious about your patterns can help you understand why you repeat certain reactions or behaviors. This creates an opportunity for healing, personal growth, and the ability to make positive changes in how we relate to others.

SECURE:

Those with this attachment style tend to have healthy communication patterns, expressing their needs and emotions openly and honestly. They are also more likely to trust their partners and feel comfortable with intimacy, fostering a solid foundation of mutual respect and understanding.

ANXIOUS-RESISTANT:

Those with this attachment style may become overly dependent on their partners for validation and reassurance. They often seek constant contact and reassurance of their partner's love and commitment. Attachment styles like this can lead to a cycle of push-pull dynamics in relationships, as they may become clingy and possessive when feeling insecure, creating tension and distance.

AVOIDANT:
Those with this attachment style may have difficulty with emotional intimacy, which can manifest in various ways, such as avoiding vulnerability or struggling to express their emotions. As a result, they may prioritize their needs and independence over their partner's, potentially leading to challenges in maintaining a deep emotional connection.

DISORGANIZED-DISORIENTED:
Those with this attachment style may struggle with trust and have difficulty forming deep emotional connections with others. Additionally, individuals with this attachment style may push people away or sabotage their relationships due to a fear of being hurt or abandoned.

Additional Practices to Increase Social Wellness

— Focus on your relationship with yourself. Compassion for ourselves resolves the separation at the root of our suffering.
— Spend some time sitting under a tree. Feeling connected to the natural world can help regulate our nervous system and calm the stress response.
— Our bodies react to the energy of others, so bringing awareness to how other people influence us is vital to our overall well-being. We can co-dysregulate just as much as we co-regulate.
— Connect with those who embody the vibration of who you want to be; people you spend time with can significantly influence your thoughts, behaviors, and personal development.
— Rekindle old friendships and nurture current, healthy relationships. If you were ever a girl Scout, you might remember the song based on a poem by Joseph Barry, "*Make new friends but keep the old; one is silver, and the other is gold.*" Sound advice that has passed the test of time.

— Practice acceptance. Self-critical thinking and judging yourself or others can hinder social interactions while keeping an open, curious mind can lead you to new relationships.

— Volunteer at an organization whose mission you respect. Doing service is a fantastic way to connect with like-minded individuals.

Remember, if you have a dysregulated nervous system, making new connections may not feel safe. Starting small while rewiring your brain for safety allows for increased connection. Additionally, seeking support from a therapist or counselor can provide valuable guidance and tools for navigating social interactions and building healthy relationships.

Practice Gratitude

Grateful people feel better about themselves and are better able to appreciate the success of others. Practicing gratitude is a simple and effective way to enhance your overall well-being and mental health. Here are some common gratitude practices you can incorporate into your daily routine:

— Morning and Evening gratitude: Begin and end your day with three things you are thankful for. This can help start and end the day positively.

—Gratitude Walk: Engage your senses and give thanks for the sights, sounds, and smells all around you.

Widen Your Circle

Join a group, take up a hobby, or enroll in a class. Meeting new people and learning new skills together is a great way to nourish your physical, intellectual, and social wellness. It is important to select activities that align with your interests and values, making the experience more enjoyable.

Try a Somatic *Check-In*

Before entering a situation that makes you feel uncomfortable, take a few minutes to check in with your body. You may notice a tightness in your body and an urge to distract yourself. As you breathe into the sensation, you may realize that the discomfort is related to a fear of rejection and vulnerability. Without judgment, acknowledge and accept you are feeling these sensations. Place your hand on the area of your body where you feel tension and sit with it-taking deep, cleansing breaths. Then, reassure yourself that even though you are anxious, you are safe. Bringing awareness and compassion to the body can help calm your nerves.

Mirror Affirmations for Deeper Self-Reflection

Gazing into a mirror enables us to connect with ourselves, mind, body, and spirit. It can boost confidence, quiet our inner critic, and help us learn to love ourselves. Mirror affirmations can be a great tool for anxiety, increased immune function, or even helping to overcome depression.

Stand in front of a mirror. Relax, take a deep, cleansing breath. Place your hands over your heart and stare into your eyes. Slowly but confidently, tell yourself affirmations that your body and mind need to hear.

I am worthy of respect and understanding.

I am strong and capable.

I am worthy of love.

I am enough.

Be aware of what comes up and sit with it without judgment. This exercise may bring up energy that is waiting to be released.

Environmental

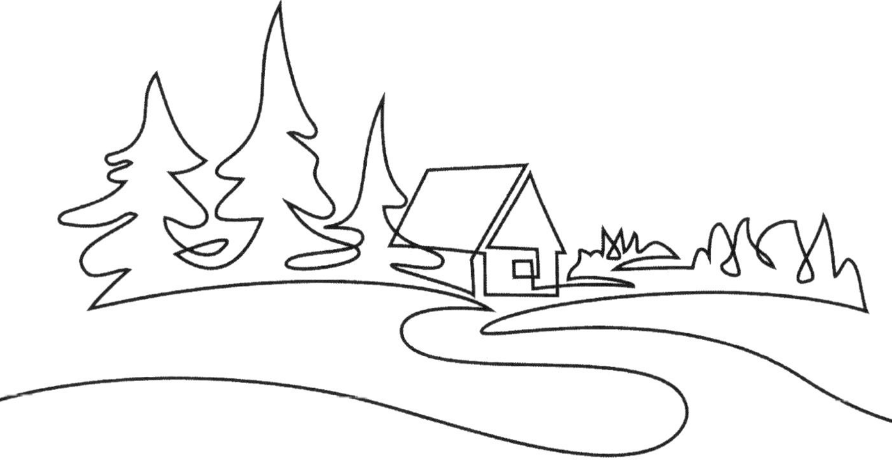

I am aware
of what sustains me
and avoid
what harms me.

“How wonderful it is that nobody needs to wait a single moment before starting to improve the world.”

—Anne Frank

Chapter 6

Environmental Wellness

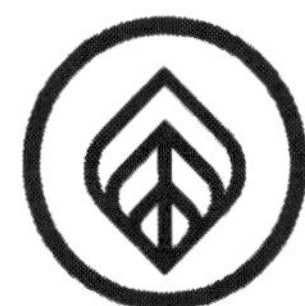

As we navigate the complexities of modern life, we yearn to uncover ways to nourish ourselves and create a harmonious balance between our inner and outer worlds. We can better understand the complex relationship between our health and our surroundings by exploring the intricate web between the two. This examination requires introspection and a willingness to explore the different aspects of our everyday lives.

We live in a fast-paced, excess-driven culture that puts a premium on short-term gratification at the expense of long-term health and happiness. We risk losing sight of what sustains us in our relentless pursuit of more. Because humans are interconnected with nature, whatever damage we are causing ourselves also affects the planet. It stands to reason that if we prioritize healing ourselves, we not only benefit personally but also contribute to a positive ripple effect in the world.

We are what we think. We are what we feel. We are what we consume. We are where we live. We are what we're exposed to. We are what we do. We are who we associate with. We become the environment in which we live. Like a mirror, our body reflects back to us, showing us the impact of our choices and behaviors. By understanding and nurturing our personal ecosystem, we can create a harmonious and thriving environment for personal growth and well-being.

> **Environmental wellness is being in tune with how our everyday life impacts us and taking responsibility for what we're exposed to in our homes, work, relationships, and greater surroundings. It is being aware of how our environment affects us and, in turn, how we affect the environment.**

Where do we start? The first step is to recognize what is causing harm to our health and well-being and then to eliminate or at least significantly reduce that harm. Although many factors are beyond our control, the choice is ours to alter what we can. Our responsibility is to foster a healthier environment for ourselves and, in turn, the planet. Changing our own habits and ways of behaving is the starting point for a better life.

> *"The way you help heal the world is you start with your own family."* —Mother Teresa

Regardless of what ails us, the remedy is to alter the equation. Modify the inputs. Transform our immediate environment. This has the potential to create a beneficial ripple effect that extends beyond our homes and into our communities. Change begins with us. By taking the initiative to make positive and lasting changes in our personal lives, we set an example for others to follow.

Be a human wellness ecologist.

Human ecology, a multidisciplinary field of study of our daily lives, seeks to demonstrate how everything we touch and are touched by is connected to our overall health. We are big fans of Daphne Miller, MD, author of *Farmacology, Total Health from the Ground Up.* Dr. Miller left her medical practice for a nationwide research project to examine what farming can teach us about nurturing and healing ourselves. How cool is that? She explains that the key to successful production is to give more attention to the farm than any particular product it may yield. A vegetable farm, for example, focuses on the soil, microbes, nutrients, and all of the farm's other components rather than the vegetables themselves.

Dr. Miller describes how the farmers she met realized that for their enterprises to survive, they needed to treat them not just as production centers but also as healthy ecosystems. Successful farmers are continuously aware of the intricate links between the farm's components. We understand why she feels that if people thought more like ecologists, we could all create profound, long-lasting changes toward better health. As we look at our "farm" (our lives), we realize that everything we surround ourselves with is somehow tied to our well-being.

Understanding ourselves as ecosystems may help us change our lives for sustainability and healing. Personal recovery then spreads like a wave to the family, community, and, eventually, the world. It all starts with us. Every one of us is responsible for taking care of and loving ourselves. We can become human wellness ecologists by experiencing life through our seven dimensions and establishing connections to how our internal and external environments impact our health and well-being.

Before considering some factors that affect our ecosystems, let's check our vitals. We live in a culture that glorifies achievement and possessions, but paradoxically, the more we have, the less satisfied we are. Food waste is plentiful, yet so many go hungry. Our nervous systems are in a constant state of fight-or-flight, and we are anxious, sick, and lonely. Our culture has become consumed with success, materialism, worry, and fear, and despite being connected 24/7, we have disconnected from each other, ourselves, and what sustains us.

We have evolved over thousands of years to seek out environments with certain qualities to satisfy our vital need for safety and security. Our environment influences our decisions and shapes our lives. It is regrettable that many of us now find it challenging to maintain a healthy balance.

According to the Centers for Disease Control (CDC), chronic disease is the leading cause of death and disability in the U.S. and costs the nation $4.1 trillion in annual healthcare costs. Six in 10 adults have a chronic disease, and four in 10 have two or more.

Life expectancy in the U.S. dropped for the second year in 2021. The decline from 77.0 to 76.1 years brought the U.S. life expectancy at birth to its lowest level since 1996.

Most people in the United States have been exposed to perfluoroalkyl and poly-fluoroalkyl substances (PFAS) or forever chemicals. Because PFAS are found in many household products, the CDC estimates that 97% of Americans have some level of PFAS in their blood. These chemicals are linked to congenital disabilities, cancer, kidney disease, liver problems, and other health issues.

Doctors are sounding the alarm that anxiety in children is skyrocketing.

Studies show obesity affects 40% of the U.S. population; almost one in four Americans had trouble affording food in 2021 (although it sounds counterintuitive, obesity and hunger are two sides of the same coin).

Our excess-obsessed culture has created an unsustainable situation. And because the planet is our mirror, everything we have done to ourselves has been done to the earth. Don't worry; we're not doom and gloom friends. Let's discuss creating a more sustainable future for ourselves and the world.

So, what sustains us?

It's time to change our thinking from what we want to what we need. Safety, nourishment, love, genuine connection, belonging, purpose, fresh air, clean water, and peace of mind. These factors influence our everyday lives and can contribute favorably or negatively to our health and well-being. As a result, becoming aware of and accepting responsibility for what we surround ourselves with at home and work, how we fuel ourselves, the quality of our relationships, and our internal thoughts are critical for wellness in this dimension.

Each of our ecological systems is unique, and listing all the possible factors influencing our everyday lives would be impossible. So, let's take a look at some common influences that can have an impact on our health and wellness. This may help spark an interest in exploring and understanding the interconnectedness between your environment and well-being.

You are what you eat.

How much thought do we give to taking care of ourselves on a daily basis? While we may not have complete control over every aspect of our lives, we influence what goes into (and onto) our bodies. Tracy was born to teach, and she delights in bringing her knowledge to life. One of her favorite experiments with kids is to demonstrate the importance of hand washing to limit the spread of germs. She begins this activity by having everyone in the class handle a freshly baked slice of bread and then rub it against different surfaces in the kitchen. The pieces are then sealed in plastic bags. Students marvel for weeks as they observe the bacteria multiply, causing the bread to develop fuzzy patches of blues and greens.

Tracy shares how one attempt at this demonstration went awry: *"The pandemic was an excellent time to rerun the experiment, but nothing happened this time—no bacterial spread, no mold at all. Instead, even after several months, the bread appeared to have just been unwrapped. What happened? Rather than homemade bread, we used a popular store-bought variety that contained calcium propionate (C.P.). C.P. is one of several additives used in processed baked goods to extend shelf life. It adds no additional value to the product. Instead, it is designed to inhibit mold growth; judging by the experiment, it works! However, research shows it can also cause headaches and damage our digestive systems. In my opinion, that's a steep price to pay for increased shelf life."*

When a headache comes on, most of us aren't wondering what ingredients were in the bread we ate for lunch. But the body knows. Chemicals like C.P. go unnoticed because most of us aren't reading labels and questioning the compounds we can't identify; we may still need to learn to make those connections. Did you know an estimated 10,000 chemicals are used in our food system? The adverse effects C.P. may have on our internal environment illustrate the potential harm these additives may cause. Since processed foods comprise a large portion of the Standard American Diet, we cannot fathom the catastrophic cumulative effect these chemicals may have on our microbiome over time. We must proactively educate ourselves about the potential dangers and make informed choices about the foods we regularly consume.

Since the beginning of time, humans have altered food to preserve it, but in modern times, we have changed some food products to the point where they no longer resemble anything found in nature. There is even a new classification for these lab-made creations: ultra-processed. We are filling our carts with addictive ultra-processed foods and getting little nourishment. As a result, we are overfed and undernourished; this is not sustainable.

"Your body responds to processed foods as if they are 'foreign bodies,' prompting an inflammatory response as it tries to protect itself."—Dr. Frank Lipman

What effect is this having on us? Evidence shows that people who eat more ultra-processed foods have a higher risk of obesity, diabetes, cardiovascular diseases, depression, cancer, and liver disease. Yet, even as awareness of the potential for harm grows, we can't seem to kick the habit. We also recognize that ultra-processed foods are cheap and sometimes the only option available to lower socioeconomic communities; studies show one in six Americans have limited access to healthy food.

Ultra-processed foods are often designed to take advantage of the brain's weaknesses, mainly how it processes pleasurable sensations. Some neuroscientists find ultra-processed foods as addictive as opioids or nicotine because they send signals to the brain's reward centers quickly and powerfully. So it makes sense why we keep returning for more. We're addicted. Although we don't believe it is our fault, making changes for our health is our responsibility.

We define "real" food as living food. Before it arrived on our plate, it was roaming the earth, swimming the seas, or growing on the farm thanks to nourishment from the soil and sun. The most nourishing and health-sustaining foods are those prepared with living food ingredients. Changing how we eat is one of the most critical steps toward enhancing our health and wellness. We recognize that change can be difficult, but becoming aware is a crucial first step!

Are the ingredients listed on the label recognizable as real food? Reading labels is an important habit to develop in order to make informed choices about the food we consume. Here is a list of some additives to avoid:

Artificial sweeteners-Aspartame (E951 - Nutrasweet or Equal) is shown to be a neurotoxin and carcinogen. It accounts for more reports of adverse reactions than all other foods and additives combined. Be aware of Acesulfame-K, a relatively new artificial sweetener. Safety testing has been called into question, and it may be linked to hormone disruption and cancer.

High fructose corn syrup (HFCS) is a refined artificial sweetener and America's number 1 source of calories. HFCS contributes to the development of diabetes and tissue damage, among other harmful effects.

MSG (Monosodium Glutamate) is an amino acid used as a flavor enhancer. MSG is an excitotoxin, a substance that overexcites cells to the point of damage or death.

Trans fat is used to enhance and extend the shelf life of food products and is among the most dangerous substances you can consume. Avoid partially hydrogenated vegetable oils.

Food dyes may contribute to children's behavioral problems and reduce I.Q. Avoid these: Blue #1 and Blue #2, Red dye # 3 and #40, Yellow #6, and Yellow Tartrazine.

Sodium sulfite is a preservative and bleaching agent that can cause congestion. The additive may play a role in the gradual disintegration of the gastrointestinal tract, particularly among those with a sensitivity.

Sodium nitrate/sodium nitrite This ingredient, which sounds harmless, is shown to be carcinogenic once it enters the human digestive system.

BHA/BHT Butylated hydroxyanisole (BHA) and butylated hydroxytoluene (BHT) are preservatives that keep foods from changing color and flavor or becoming rancid. They may affect the brain's neurological system, alter behavior, and may cause cancer.

Sulfur dioxide (E220) is an additive used in the food and drinks industries for its properties as a preservative and antioxidant. It may be detrimental to the respiratory system and linked to cardiovascular disease.

Potassium bromate is an additive used to increase the volume of some white flour, bread, and rolls; potassium bromate is known to cause animal cancer. Even small amounts may create problems for humans.

It should be emphasized that while we are not to blame for toxic ingredients, we do need to educate ourselves and limit our consumption. It is imperative to slow down and pay attention to how we nourish ourselves; we cannot thrive in an environment that makes us sick. Real food is nutrient-rich and essential for our survival. Start today with simple changes!

While we understand that manufacturers are working toward their bottom line, many of them are the most significant contributors to our global health crisis. Therefore, it is essential to educate ourselves on the impact of our choices. Doing so can create a demand for sustainable and healthy products, positively impacting our health and the environment.

Of course, none of this addresses accessibility; food deserts are places where residents cannot access healthy, affordable food. We are still learning how to be better allies and agents of change. However, one potential solution to address accessibility is to support local farmers and community gardens, which can provide fresh produce to areas lacking grocery store access. Additionally, advocating for policy changes and increased funding for programs promoting healthy food options in underserved communities can have a significant impact. Let's work together to build a system where responsibly grown, nutrient-dense food is available to all.

Seeing skin as a way IN.

Picture this: the average American woman uses around 12 personal care items every day, totaling 168 different chemicals. The majority of these substances come into direct contact with our skin, the body's largest organ, which allows them to be absorbed into the bloodstream.

It's time to don the cape of knowledge! Educating ourselves about the potential perils lurking in certain products is our superhero move. Armed with information, we can make choices that whisper, "I care about my health," and take charge of what we slather and spray on ourselves. Certain chemicals in cosmetics, sunscreens, and personal care items can impact the endocrine system, disrupting hormone production and regulation. This disruption has been linked to various health issues, including reproductive problems, immune system dysfunction, and cancer.

Enter two of our favorite guardians of consumer safety: Valisure and the Environmental Working Group (EWG)! They're the unsung heroes, playing a significant role in advocating for consumer safety and transparency. EWG provides valuable tools, including the Clean 15 and Dirty Dozen, to help consumers make informed choices about the products we use. Check out their impressive database for safer personal care products!

Meet Valisure, the independent testing lab from New Haven, CT, where Harvard- and Yale-trained scientists unite. They're not afraid to wield their testing powers and uncover critical issues. Imagine this: they found benzene (a well-documented Group 1 carcinogen and environmental hazard) in 27% of the over 600 sunscreen and after-sun products they tested. This information is imperative for our well-being and underscores the importance of independent testing.

By staying informed and making conscious choices, we can drive the demand for safer products and encourage companies to prioritize consumer health. Additionally, supporting organizations like Valisure and EWG helps to hold manufacturers accountable and push for stricter regulations in the personal care industry. Together, we have the power to create a safer and healthier future for ourselves and future generations.

Social media: The drama dilemma.

Let's switch gears and talk about the digital rollercoaster known as social media. Social wellness reminds us that humans are wired for connection and seek out meaningful relationships. We need connection to thrive, and social media can help us feel closer to others. Or so it seems. Shankar Vedantam, in Diane's favorite newsletter, Hidden Brain, from February 2023 (seriously, check out his podcast!), wonders: If social media were more sociable, would we be as glued to it? Contrary to common sense, social media's toxic nature might be one of its draws.

The newsletter quotes a recent study that found that people are more likely to engage with negative or controversial content on social media platforms. This suggests that the addictive nature of social media may stem from our desire for drama and conflict rather than genuine connection. In other words, while social media platforms have the potential to bring people together, they may also be fueling our fascination with negativity and controversy. In order to break free from this cycle, it is important to be mindful of our online behavior and actively seek out positive and uplifting content that promotes genuine social interaction.

Here's the tea: even if we use social media accounts to feel connected, there is evidence that frequent usage is associated with an elevated threat of isolation, anxiety, depression, and self-harm. Always keep in mind that genuine connection is what sustains us. By prioritizing meaningful connections and seeking out positive content, we can create a healthier online environment for ourselves and others. Need a breather? Take a digital detox and savor real-life moments to keep our social and emotional well-being in check. Ultimately, it is up to us to use social media mindfully and in moderation. This is your invitation to call a friend or loved one, have a face-to-face conversation, and strengthen those personal connections.

Assessing and Addressing Unhealthy Relationships.

"I beg to differ" is how Tracy introduced herself to her best friend when they first met at a book club. For over 20 years, they have challenged each other to think critically and more broadly. Relationships don't always have to be agreeable, but they should be based on respect and genuine care for one another. Spending time with others should make you feel more connected and give you energy, not drain it.

Paying attention to our bodies when we're around people can be telling; remember, the body is our barometer. Are you left with a feeling of "YES"? Or do you frequently experience an unsettling sensation that alerts you to a misalignment? The body knows.

When you're in a relationship that isn't healthy, it's critical to set personal boundaries about what you won't stand for. If that person consistently disregards your boundary lines, it may be time to reassess your position. Ending toxic relationships can be challenging and sometimes dangerous. If you find yourself in this situation, seek the help of a professional to help you explore the best options for you.

"You cannot have a positive life with a negative mind."
—Joyce Meyer

We tend to think of toxins as poisonous substances, but toxins can be defined as anything that impedes well-being. For example, we talk to ourselves more than anyone else, and negative self-talk can be just as harmful to our bodies as poisonous substances. In discussing taking control of our thoughts, three notable examples come to mind: Louie Zamperini, prisoner of war; Victor Frankl, holocaust survivor and author of *Man's Search for Meaning*; and Nelson Mandela, who went from prisoner to the first black president of South Africa.

Amid horrific conditions, each individual chose not to be a victim of circumstance. Frankl shares his incredible will to survive the concentration camp: "Every day, every hour, offered the opportunity to make a decision, a decision which determined whether you would or would not submit to those powers which threatened to rob you of your very self, your inner freedom, which determined whether or not you would become the plaything of circumstance."

Although we may not always control our environment, we can always direct our thoughts. Rewiring our brains toward a growth mindset can help us overcome even the most difficult challenges in life.

Is messiness messing with me?

Even though accumulating "stuff" might not seem like a big deal, since our homes are extensions of our energy fields, clutter can harm our mental health. We may experience heaviness, imbalance, and immobility when there is a disorder in the form of clutter. It may also be surprising to learn that it can raise stress levels and damage relationships.

"When your environment is clean, you feel happy, motivated, and healthy." —Lailah Gifty Akita

The good news is that organizing our environment and creating space can similarly impact our minds. This idea aligns with the principles of environmental psychology and the connection between our surroundings and mental well-being. According to Stephanie Bennet Vogt, leading space clearing expert, teacher, and author, spaciousness is not something we do or get or study for, but rather a quality of being that we cultivate, and it can lead us to personal transformation and freedom. Make room for the life you want.

Stephanie's practices help us regulate our brain's fight-or-flight responses and ease us into new routines that feel good and result in long-lasting change. But first, we need awareness and consistency, which means practicing daily. One example is to get a broom and sweep a room, a floor, or any cobwebs that are difficult to reach. Cleaning can be used as a metaphor to create a new beginning. Every day, sweep a small portion of your home and observe its impact on your nervous system and mindset.

Do something today that your future self will thank you for.

A well-rounded existence begins with the conscious investment of time and energy into making one's own surroundings healthier and more sustainable. We can improve our daily choices by practicing mindfulness and consciously connecting our inputs and actions to our outcomes.

Reconnecting with nature is critical for individual and environmental health. It's not a coincidence that people find healing in nature when experiencing difficult times. Studies have shown that spending time outdoors positively affects our physical and emotional well-being. In times of strife, life often slows down enough for us to see the link. But don't wait for those times! Make it a priority to spend time in nature regularly, whether walking in the park or hiking in the mountains. Not only will it enhance our quality of life, but it will also help cultivate a deeper appreciation and respect for the environment.

New research shows that diet, stress, exercise, exposure to toxic food, air and water, electromagnetic radiation, and trauma may affect our genes. Dr. Mark Hyman, physician, author, founder, and medical director of The UltraWellness Center, reminds us why improving environmental factors is connected to living our best lives. Although our genes may predispose us to certain diseases, our DNA is not a set blueprint.

Dr. Hyman asserts that improving these environmental elements can change how our bodies respond. In other words, we may not be able to alter our genes, but we can modify how our environment interacts with them. We can take control of our health and create better futures for ourselves by incorporating simple, positive changes into our everyday lives.

Remember, what sustains us is safety, nourishment, genuine connection, love, belonging, purpose, fresh air, clean water, and peace of mind. We would be remiss not to add equity and justice to that list. By being ambassadors of healing, love, and kindness, we can spark change toward creating an environment that honors all members of our greater community.

When we take responsibility for bringing healing to ourselves, we encourage and inspire those around us to do the same. And because we are mirrors of nature, healing ourselves can impact the environment's recovery. Never underestimate the ripple effect one small change can make. It starts with us.

With the realization that everything we touch or are touched by relates in some way to our well-being, what simple shifts can you make toward a more sustainable future?

"By cleansing your body on a regular basis and eliminating as many toxins as possible from your environment, your body can begin to heal itself, prevent disease, and become stronger and more resilient than you ever dreamed possible."
– Dr. Edward Group III, CEO of Global Healing Center

IT'S AN INSIDE JOB:
Practices for self-regulation

The body has a limited ability to detoxify. Our detoxification capacity is unique to each of us. How can you tell when you are having trouble handling your toxic load? Your body will tell you! But you have to pay attention and make the connection. Increased awareness helps us make informed choices. Here are a few of the most common symptoms that may appear when our detox systems become overwhelmed:

— Headaches and migraines
— Constipation or diarrhea
— Inflammatory skin conditions
— Joint or muscle pain
— Weight gain
— Fatigue
— Insomnia
— Depression
— Brain fog or trouble concentrating
— Sinus problems
— Swollen gums
— Sore throat

You may notice that these symptoms can mimic other conditions. If your symptoms don't pass or your condition worsens, it's essential to seek medical advice.

To get a feel for how your environmental factors may affect your body's internal mechanisms, try the following and be aware of any changes:

Do LESS of this:

x Eat ultra-processed foods
x Clean with dangerous chemicals
x Use skincare products made with toxic compounds
x Drink your calories
x Tune into news and social media
x Consume foods with high fructose corn syrup or artificial sweeteners
x Use non-stick cookware
x Buy single-use products
x Negative thinking
x Frequent use of electronics
x Consumption of alcohol and caffeine
x Plastic water bottles and containers

And MORE of this:

— Move your body
— Foster healthy relationships
— Wash your produce
— Drink a lot of clean, filtered water
— Eat whole foods. Go organic and local when possible
— Support the liver with herbs like dandelion, turmeric, and milk thistle
— Practice a growth mindset
— Get quality sleep
— Practice deep breathing exercises
— Get outside!

Occupational

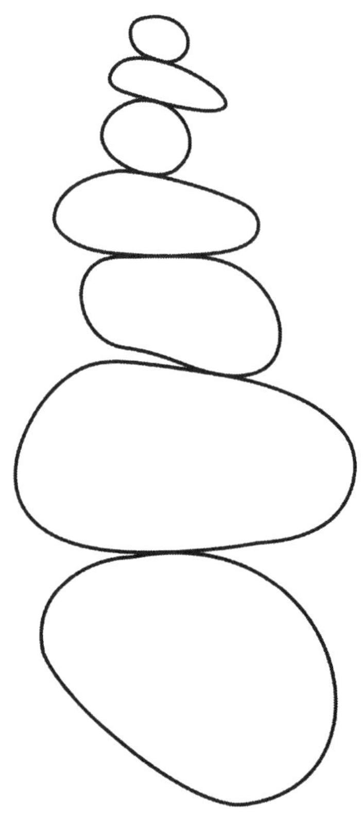

I am purposeful
and seek satisfaction
in what I do.

"People used to ask me what I wanted to be when I grew up and I'd say "Happy!" That was all I wanted to be."

—Goldie Hawn

Chapter 7

Occupational Wellness

What do you want to be when you grow up? This question is posed to almost every young person at some point during their formative years. Working with teens has taught us that this can sometimes feel like pressure. Teens often feel overwhelmed by the expectation of a clear career path, especially when they are still discovering their passions and interests. It's important to remember that the journey of self-discovery and career exploration is ongoing, even for adults.

What if we change the dialogue to ask open-ended questions, all while reassuring our youth that we will love them regardless of the career path they choose? What if we ask what sparks curiosity? What do you want to learn? Would it change their direction and, more importantly, their happiness? Or imagine the outcome if we guide them toward what inspires them instead of emphasizing achievement. They may see that their life has meaning beyond a title or paycheck.

Occupational wellness is gaining personal fulfillment from a job, career, or volunteer position while still maintaining balance in life.

Similar to other dimensions, bringing awareness to our childhood experiences can connect us to hidden beliefs that may affect our abilities and satisfaction in the workplace. With a curious lens, try to connect your childhood experiences with your current behavior and work styles. If you were raised in an environment where hard work and success were highly valued, you may have developed a strong drive to excel. If work was a means to an end in your household, you might struggle with finding purpose and fulfillment in your professional life. Was achievement seen as the only path to success? These questions might reveal how your upbringing shaped your mindset and attitude toward work.

Understanding these influences can help us make conscious decisions to chart a course that aligns with our values and goals. By recognizing the impact of our childhood experiences, we can work toward breaking any negative patterns or beliefs that may have been ingrained in us and embrace positive aspects with intentionality. This self-awareness allows us to challenge and redefine our own definitions of success and happiness.

Let's investigate the influence a mother can have on her daughter's career potential. In the working paper *Children and Gender Inequality: Evidence From Denmark* by Henrik Kleven, Camille Landais, and Jakob Egholt Søgaard, the authors found that women whose mothers worked outside the home were more likely to have higher aspirations and pursue careers. This suggests that positive role models can significantly impact a woman's success. Furthermore, the study also reveals that women with working mothers were more likely to have higher earnings and hold leadership positions in their careers.

"When I grow up, I want to be an old woman."
—Michelle Shocked

We also wanted to know how working parents affected their children's mental health. To answer that question, we turned to a study by Stewart D. Friedman, an organizational psychologist at the Wharton School, and Jeff Greenhaus from Drexel University. In a *Harvard Business Review* article, Friedman explains that their research examined the relationship between parental career choices and children's mental health outcomes.

Friedman says, "We found that children's emotional health was higher when parents believed that family should come first, regardless of how much time they spent working. We also found children were better off when parents cared about work as a source of challenge, creativity, and enjoyment, again, without regard to the time spent. And, not surprisingly, we saw that children were better off when parents were able to be physically available to them."

We asked Diane to share her story to help bring this topic to life:

"I am child number four of eight; my mother was a stay-at-home mom. My family dynamics limited my options when it came to furthering my education. However, this did not hold me back; I created a self-directed educational journey, became a lifelong learner, and, along the way, found fulfillment in three different careers.

When my first child was born, I began reacting to an internalized belief that 'good mothers' do not work outside the home. So, when my second child was born, I left my job as a branch manager at a bank. I thought being home was what was expected of me, and my career took a back seat for a few years.

In my thirties, my father died, and I got a divorce. The decade was an emotional roller coaster, but my grief and transition propelled me forward.

I returned to the workplace through this challenging period and stepped into 'my power.'

I have been a stay-at-home mom, a mom who worked outside the home part-time, and a single mom who worked 40+ hours a week regularly. When my kids were little, I often worried I worked too many hours. I feared they would resent the time I spent away from them. My mother's choice not to work outside the home impacted me when I first entered the workforce; however, today, I don't think there is a right or wrong answer. Research shows that parents who work in a positive environment are more likely to have positive experiences outside of work. What seemed to matter most to the well-being of my family was the energy, love, and balance I brought back into the home.

We must each choose what is best for our financial and emotional well-being. Having a successful work life while creating a loving home life gave my children the 'permission' to grow and succeed themselves. Although my children are now grown, it remains critically important to me that I work in a healthy environment.

Of course, work matters because it allows us to support ourselves, be purposeful, and see ourselves as part of something bigger than ourselves. But what matters most is its impact on our overall well-being. Work provides us with fulfillment and accomplishment, helping us develop our skills and talents. The awareness that the environment we work in can impact every dimension of our lives can help us stand in our power, make changes when necessary, and choose the right path for us."

I am the measure of my worth. I am worthy.

It may be a new concept to think about self-love in the workplace. When we prioritize our well-being and treat ourselves with kindness, it can increase productivity, improve relationships with colleagues, and give us greater fulfillment in our work. Additionally, understanding the connection between our nervous system, belief system, and mindset can help us better manage stress and respond more effectively to challenges in the workplace. We need to differentiate between self-esteem, self-worth, and self-love. They do sound similar, but each contributes differently to our wellness in this dimension.

Self-esteem is our confidence level in our worth; it describes how we think and feel about ourselves. It can be very fluid, changing based on our circumstances, mood, or how others make us feel.

Self-worth has more depth; it is the stable, comprehensive way we look at ourselves. Strong self-worth is the belief that we are loveable and valuable regardless of how we view our skills and traits. It comes from self-love, knowing and believing in our worth.

Self-love means we fully accept all aspects of our being. We treat ourselves with kindness, respect, and compassion and have a high regard for our happiness and well-being.

So, let's look at three examples of how these can play out in a work setting. For each illustration, assume that your boss has asked that you present a new concept for management to consider.

Example 1: At the beginning of the meeting, when you prepare to speak, your heart begins to race, and your anxiety is in full swing. Your voice is shaky, and you have very little confidence while presenting. Fortunately, everyone loves the idea, so your self-esteem picks up during the meeting. However, after the meeting, you beat yourself up with negative self-talk. You feel you weren't qualified to be in the meeting; everyone is more capable than you. *What happened?* Your self-esteem fluctuated; you had low self-worth and did not show yourself love.

Example 2: At the beginning of the meeting, when you prepare to speak, your heart begins to race, and your anxiety is in full swing. You take a deep, cleansing breath before you start. You are composed and confident as you present. Unfortunately, no one likes your idea; your new concept is rejected. When the meeting ends, your self-esteem is very low, and you question your abilities in this role. But you take another cleansing breath and tell yourself you still have value. *What happened?* By taking deep breaths, you were practicing self-regulation. Of course, your self-esteem fluctuated based on the outcome, but your self-worth carried you through.

Example 3: At the beginning of the meeting, when you prepare to speak, your heart begins to race, and your anxiety is in full swing. You take a deep cleansing breath and say, "Hello, Anxiety, I see you, but step aside—I got this." You are composed, confident, and relaxed as you present. Unfortunately, no one likes your idea; your new concept is shut down. When the meeting ended, you asked for feedback; what specifically about the idea didn't you like? How could I have performed better? *What happened?* Your mind stayed on task because you used two self-regulating tools (deep breaths and befriending resistance). As a result, both your self-esteem and your self-worth remained steady. Then, you used a growth mindset to accept feedback with a willingness to learn and grow.

When we bring awareness to ourselves, we can better understand our reactions and make improvements. By seeking feedback and reflecting on the situation, we can gain valuable insights into what went wrong and how to improve for future presentations. Additionally, embracing a growth mindset allows you to see failure as an opportunity for growth rather than a reflection of your worth or abilities.

Finding fulfillment and balance.

Whether at a job or a volunteer position, occupational wellness is about finding fulfillment and satisfaction in what we do. As we delve further into this dimension, let's focus on what these qualities feel like inside our bodies. Try a little self-exploration: How do I feel on my way to work? Do

I feel supported and valued when I'm at work? Is my body tense at work or when thinking about my job? Do I feel anxiety when Sunday rolls around? How do I feel after a few days off? By paying attention to our physical and emotional responses to work, we can make adjustments to create a more balanced experience.

"Never get so busy making a living that you forget to make a life." —Dolly Parton

Hardly anyone made it through the pandemic without impacting their occupational wellness. Many individuals experienced changes in their work environment, whether transitioning to remote work, facing a job loss, or juggling kids at home. Some awoke to realize they had been barely surviving for years while calling it life. These shifts forced people to reevaluate their priorities and consider the importance of finding fulfillment and balance in their careers. Throughout America, COVID-19 brought to life terms like great resignation and quiet quitting.

Quiet quitting refers to mentally disengaging from our jobs while still physically showing up to work. It is a silent resignation that can lead to emptiness and dissatisfaction in one's professional life. As people become more aware of the negative effects of silently quitting, they are recognizing the importance of finding meaning and balance in their careers. Prioritizing self-care, setting boundaries, and exploring new opportunities can help us break free from the cycle of quiet quitting and rediscover passion and purpose in our professional lives.

Making a change can be scary and uncertain, but it can also be a transformative experience that leads to personal growth and fulfillment. We asked Helen to share her experience navigating the pandemic while trusting her intuition to pursue a new career.

"Like many others, the pandemic negatively impacted my overall well-being, including social, emotional, and occupational wellness. COVID happened as I was making a career change from working in Art Production & Design. I was beginning to feel physically and emotionally stuck, and I knew I needed to find a new path.

After some (okay, a lot!) of self-exploration, I returned to school for my Master's in Counseling. I knew continuing my education would positively impact my occupational wellness, and the timing was such that it kept me busy and engaged with the outside world (via Zoom). The decision fed my brain and relieved some of my dis-ease.

People often ask why I went from the New York City design and publishing world to counseling in Connecticut. They are perceived to be two different worlds, both geographically and occupationally. But that's not how I see it. My life experiences led me to this moment. I love publishing; it's an extension of who I am. It was a great career, but something deep inside told me I was ready for a change.

Connecting with someone who is struggling with something that I understand and offering them connection, hope, and tools for healing gives me a deep feeling of fulfillment. This book is another extension of who I am. The content is about our collective experiences. It's about creating good in the world and discovering who we are each meant to be. I feel blessed that I found the inner strength to listen to those needs."

Does being busy all the time put us on the road to success?

Being busy, once seen as a badge of honor, can hinder our ability to find happiness and satisfaction in our lives. With deeper exploration, it can sometimes be seen as a trauma response—keeping ourselves in overdrive can be a way of avoiding what we are subconsciously afraid of. If we don't slow down, we don't have to be present, and we won't have to feel. We all have different stress thresholds, so what constitutes "too busy" for one may differ for another. Bringing awareness to how our body reacts to stress will help us understand the risks of being overworked all the time. Stress is at the root of many physical, mental, and relational issues that result from being overly busy.

> *"Productivity is not how much work I do in a day but how well I balance what I need to stay healthy. Being productive is knowing when to rest."* —Rupi Kaur

As outlined in the first chapter, the stress response is the body's defense system. When the nervous system detects a threat, it triggers the release of stress hormones such as cortisol and adrenaline. These hormones prepare the body by boosting heart rate, blood pressure, and alertness. When we are constantly in a state of stress due to being overly busy, our bodies remain in this heightened state for prolonged periods of time. As humans, we are not designed to be under constant stress. Ignoring the need for rest and relaxation can result in a weakened immune system, burnout, and career damage. Self-awareness and self-worth are needed to help us recognize when to step back and evaluate our situation. It's important to note we can make the best decisions for ourselves when we can see our worth outside of the context of our jobs.

Emotional exhaustion is the number one sign of burnout, according to Dr. Ricky Fernandez, PT, DPT, Burnout Coach. This crippling sense of exhaustion is frequently a result of ongoing stress in one's work and personal environment. Burnout sufferers may become cynical about their work as their jobs become more stressful. At the same time, they might begin to lose interest in their work and become less emotionally invested; their performance often decreases. According to a 2021 study conducted by Oracle and Workplace Intelligence, an HR research and advisory firm, 75% of respondents feel professionally trapped, and 29% said they are struggling financially. But, maybe most alarming is that 28% indicated they suffer from worsening mental health, and 23% feel detached from their own lives. These findings highlight the urgent need for organizations to address and mitigate burnout in order to support their employees' holistic well-being.

We met Janice at a volunteer opportunity that brings people together in service to others. It is a unique environment created and held in the energy of love. The organization is a magnet to countless volunteers seeking purpose and belonging; a sense of safety allows for vulnerability and genuine connection among volunteers and staff. So we were initially saddened when, after only a few months, Janice announced she was leaving, closing her shop and moving south. Janice owned a salon and had been in business for many years but reported being unhappy for the last decade. Chronic stress affected her health, marriage, and how she wanted to show up in the world. However, Janice shared that spending a few hours each week in a safe and connected environment allowed her to tap into her intuition; something inside called her to a better life. Returning to herself, she could finally permit herself to leave. Watching Janice reconnect with her inner knowing and step into her power was inspiring.

Put yourself on top of your to-do list.

We understand not everyone can walk away from their job; a January 2023 survey by LendingClub indicates that 60% of consumers say they're living paycheck to paycheck. That being said, we can permit ourselves to explore other options if we sense a need for a change, especially in cases where our workplace is toxic. It shouldn't be considered a failure or quitting when our job causes physical, mental, or emotional harm. Taking care of ourselves should always be a priority, and sometimes that means making difficult decisions for our own well-being. It's important to remember that our job does not define our worth, and finding a healthier environment can lead to a better life.

Finding a sense of purpose outside of work can be very satisfying if we know our job is a means to an end and leaving isn't an option. This could involve pursuing hobbies, volunteering, or building meaningful relationships outside work. Remember that our worth goes beyond employment, and finding meaning and satisfaction in one of our other dimensions may help us improve our well-being and happiness. You matter. Let's move you to the top of the list.

EQ and you.

In our experience, authenticity, and safety are crucial to company culture. Employees should feel comfortable expressing their thoughts and concerns without fear of retribution. This fosters a sense of trust and belonging within the organization, ultimately leading to increased productivity and employee satisfaction. It is important for leaders to prioritize emotional intelligence (EQ) and actively work towards creating a supportive and inclusive work environment.

Diane's introduction to the concept of EQ came from Deb, one of her managers and a long-time mentor. Deb recommended reading "*Emotional Intelligence: Why It Can Matter More Than IQ*" by Daniel Goleman, Ph.D., and they later had a thoughtful discussion about the book. Despite being crafted as a managerial tool, they both acknowledged that emotional intelligence holds equal significance for employees. The five key elements of high EQ are beneficial for both leaders and employees to portray:

Self-awareness is demonstrated by identifying and understanding how emotions and actions can impact those around you. Both leaders and

employees with high EQ clearly understand their strengths and weaknesses.
Self-regulation is demonstrated by maintaining calm and controlling emotions. Both leaders and employees with high EQ regulate themselves effectively and take responsibility for their actions.
Motivation is demonstrated by the ability to drive toward objectives of our own volition versus external expectations or rewards.
Empathy is demonstrated by understanding others from a place of compassion; this is crucial to developing trust within the team and between the group and leadership.
Social skills are demonstrated by communicating well and making genuine connections. Leaders and team members with high EQ are diplomatic in times of conflict and manage change well; they are able to give praise freely and sincerely.

Recently, Diane had the opportunity to have dinner and catch up with Deb, whom she now considers a good friend. While discussing "the good old days," Deb said something that opened Diane's eyes and made her understand why she is a fantastic leader. Paraphrasing Deb's words, "I sometimes wondered how we got so much work done. When we allowed people to be authentic at work, they showed up with their traumas, stumbling blocks, knowledge, and skills. Somehow, I accomplished more when I sat with people and actively listened to their stories."

By allowing people to bring their whole selves to work, Deb created an environment where individuals felt comfortable sharing their experiences and ideas. This fostered a sense of trust and camaraderie among the team and allowed for a deeper understanding of each person's unique strengths and challenges. As a result, Deb was able to tap into the full potential of her team and achieve remarkable results.

While emotional intelligence is crucial for good management, employees with high EQ thrive in the workplace. They are more self-aware, can handle challenging situations more efficiently, form strong bonds, and have high leadership potential. Moreover, these individuals are often seen as reliable and trustworthy, as they prioritize honesty and integrity in their interactions. Overall, their high EQ not only benefits their own personal growth but also enhances the overall success of the organization.

Embracing an entrepreneurial mindset.

Self-employment gives us the autonomy and control to prioritize tasks on our to-do lists. This can lead to a better work-life balance and the ability to pursue passions outside of work. With just a slight mental adjustment, we can see that even employees who are not self-employed are working for themselves. By taking ownership of our work and seeing it as a reflection of us, we can find fulfillment and satisfaction in our jobs.

According to author and leadership executive/coach Bill Abatte, a shift happens when we adopt an entrepreneurial mindset. To embrace this concept, Bill advises visualizing ourselves working for our own company, "You, Inc." Entrepreneurs often have a growth mindset, embracing lifelong learning and self-improvement. Although an employer may hire us directly, we sell them our knowledge and services. It can be for the short term or the long term, just like any business that offers a service to other companies. In today's society, we'll probably sell our services to several companies over a lifetime. Just as businesses build their brand and reputation, we can develop a personal brand. This brand should reflect our unique skills, experience, and expertise.

Most recently, those entering the workforce seem to have taken on the idea naturally and, in many ways, have changed the workplace. With this subtle shift in perspective, we can prioritize balance and more easily uphold our values, increasing our job satisfaction.

Get out the map.

Goals are very important to us because they give us a sense of meaning and direction. They are like lighthouses that illuminate the way to success in both our personal and professional lives. Setting clear goals gives us a blueprint for our journey and helps us focus our energy on specific goals. This focus helps us direct efforts effectively, avoid distractions, and make choices that are in line with our desired outcomes.

Goals basically push us forward by giving us a clear picture of what we want to achieve. Moreover, they contribute significantly to personal growth and development. In order to reach our goals, we often have to push ourselves beyond our comfort zones. This process of challenging oneself to do more makes us more resilient, flexible and always looking for ways to improve. Setting goals also allows us to measure our progress and celebrate achievements along the way.

On the road to success.

Tuning into the health of our nervous system can allow us to manage stress better and keep us from burning out at work. This involves paying attention to physical and emotional cues, practicing self-care activities such as exercise and mindfulness, and seeking support when needed. By prioritizing self-awareness in the workplace, we can enhance our ability to make informed decisions, navigate challenges effectively, and build meaningful personal and professional relationships. Investing in ourselves is not selfish but essential to achieving long-term success and happiness.

By shifting our focus from attaining external milestones to prioritizing personal growth and fulfillment, we can cultivate a more harmonious and holistic approach to success. This shift in perspective allows us to embrace the journey and focus on how we want to show up in the workplace. It helps us prioritize our professional objectives alongside our well-being and outside relationships by encouraging us to establish limits and achieve a healthy work-life balance.

Right now, the project is YOU! We need to invest time and effort in understanding ourselves, identifying our strengths and weaknesses, and setting clear goals for personal and professional growth. When we view ourselves as an ongoing work in progress, we can grow, change, and develop at our own pace, setting ourselves up for success. Remember, success is not solely defined by our professional achievements but also by the satisfaction and joy we bring to all aspects of our lives.

Decide what matters to you. Who do you want to be? Set attainable goals, work on improving yourself, ensure your efforts align with your values, and celebrate small wins along the way. You got this!

"To laugh often and much:
To win the respect of intelligent people
and the affection of children,
to earn the appreciation of honest critics
and endure the betrayal of false friends;
to appreciate beauty, to find the best in others,
to leave the world a bit better
whether by a healthy child, a garden patch,
or a redeemed social condition;
to know even one life has breathed easier because you lived.
This is to have succeeded."
—Ralph Waldo Emerson

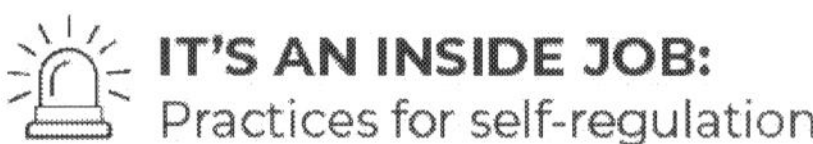

EQ allows us to thrive in the workplace. Being more aware of our earliest experiences and having a sense of self-worth makes finding balance and personal satisfaction possible.

Who Do You Want to Be When You Grow Up?

Okay, we know you're a grown-up, but don't let that stop you from growing. Be curious. It doesn't matter what you do or accomplish; what matters is how you show up. Who do you want to BE? Exploring this from a fresh perspective can help you gain perspective and deeper satisfaction.

Be Curious About Your Leadership Style.

Your first leadership role models were most likely your parents or caregivers. What kind of leaders were they? Did their guidance and decision-making skills influence your own leadership style? How did they set boundaries? How did they show you love? Bringing awareness to what initially shaped your perceptions and how they influenced your leadership style can help you become a more effective leader and team member.

Reflect on instances where you observed your parents demonstrate leadership qualities and how that impacted your perception of leadership.

Remember how your parents established limits with you as a child and the idea of boundaries in leadership. Were these strategies successful?

Examine the role of love in leadership, drawing from personal experiences. It is essential to recognize that love in leadership does not mean being soft or weak but instead being able to connect with and inspire others through genuine understanding.

Burnout Early Warning Signs May Include:

— Emotional exhaustion
— Headaches or gastrointestinal upset
— Trouble sleeping
— Anxiety
— Brain fog that results in difficulty concentrating
— An inability to have meaningful connections with others
— Irritability and black-and-white thinking

Ways to Reduce Workplace Stress.

Free up mental space to enable better focus and productivity:
Walk at lunch to help clear the mind and gain greater perspective. Taking a break and engaging in physical activity can increase focus, and boost energy levels, leading to better performance in the workplace.
Explore yoga, tai chi, or chi gong to move with calm, stillness, and breath in the face of challenges. Incorporate these ancient practices into your routine to foster balance and a growth mindset.
Observe your internal dialogue to avoid counter-productive self-criticism. Treat yourself with the same kindness and understanding that you would a good friend.
Meditate for a few minutes during your workday. Taking time to clear your mind and focus on your breath can help reduce stress and improve productivity throughout the day.
Play reduces stress and boosts health. While working together at a wellness organization, Diane made carrot costumes, and Tracy eagerly volunteered to be a carrot for a company event—check out her picture in the back of the book!

Spiritual

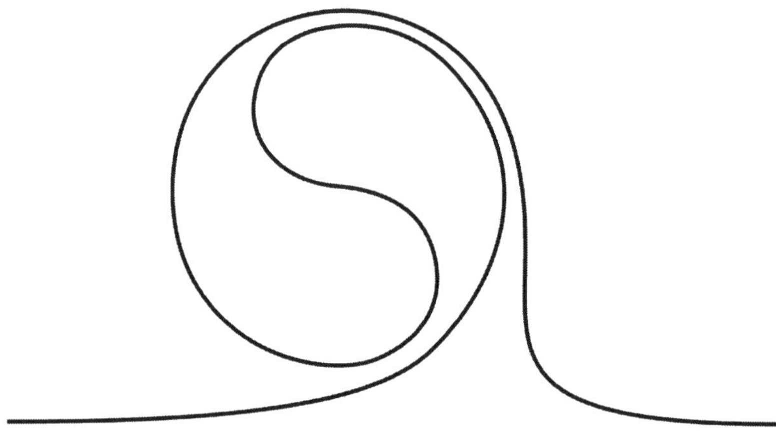

I am love
and I share
my gifts with
the world.

“I am because we are.”

—The African Philosophy of Ubuntu

Chapter 8

Spiritual Wellness

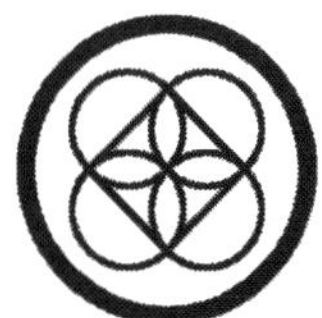

A big belly laugh, a warm smile, or a sorrowful tear can transcend language barriers and connect us on a cellular level. Spirituality is a universal language, allowing us to feel a sense of belonging and to connect with something greater than ourselves. Regardless of our individual beliefs or backgrounds, spirituality can unite us in a shared experience of the human condition. It is our restorative journey.

When we first started conceptualizing this dimension, we sought out friends for different perspectives, only to discover that a number of them were completely opposed to contributing to this chapter. We were reminded that spirituality is a sensitive topic. Each appeared to be on a path of deconditioning—looking for significance outside of their upbringing or searching for a higher purpose. It isn't lost on any of us that this "search" is deeply spiritual. We appreciate and respect each person's unique and highly personal path toward finding meaning and purpose.

Spiritual wellness is our deepest level of consciousness. It is the state of being connected to something greater than ourselves, and finding meaning and purpose in life.

As we deepened the conversation, we came up with other ways to describe "spirit," such as God, soul, heart, universe, life force, inner light, and true essence. Wherever you are on your journey, we hope you come to see, as we have, that there is a unique but similar essence in each of us. What we are searching for can be found inside of us.

Ponder this: Who is the listener after comprehending that the mind is a system? Who is there to observe the thinker? The listener is our inner self. We learn that our ideas, emotions, and bodies are constantly shifting and changing, but there is a witness within us that doesn't change—our spirit. Our spirit uses the mind and body to experience the outside world.

"You don't have a soul. You are a soul. You have a body."
—C.S. Lewis

Children serve as one of the best reminders of who we really are. They see the world through the eyes of wonder and opportunity. A child can see a palace in a refrigerator box or transform a simple bath towel into a superhero's cape. Watching children filled with curiosity and joy, we see our true essence. The same joyful life force that delights in the simplest of things is also within us. It is a reminder that we, too, have the ability to find joy and wonder in our everyday lives, if only we choose to embrace it. In effect, whenever we are immersed in the present moment, we experience the expansive and timeless nature of the spirit.

Just as the body is the barometer for well-being, the soul is the glue that holds our dimensions together. We all have access to deep feelings of love, hope, kindness, compassion, empathy, wonder, possibility, and awe for everything we hold sacred. Spirituality also means being conscious of the opposite parts of ourselves. Part of spiritual growth is becoming aware of and accepting our shadows. Being genuine and showing up as our complete selves is crucial to our experience here on Earth.

What if it's that simple? What if it's about authenticity? What if it's about Love? What if recognizing and accepting our whole selves while sharing love in our own ways is why we are here?

We understand that each of us is on a different spiritual path, and we hope you will continue to read this chapter with an open heart. Hearing others' stories allows us to gain deeper insights into our journeys and helps expand our definition of what it means to be spiritual. Using a growth mindset will assist us in being open to the experiences of others, even when they are different from our own.

Finding and loving ourselves.

Our paths to personal development are unique and winding, and they all require time. Each of us possesses innate qualities and unique talents that, when nurtured, can lead us to a life filled with purpose and fulfillment. However, the journey of life, with its external influences, challenging events, and moments of self-doubt, can sometimes overshadow these natural inclinations and shape our perceptions of ourselves and the world. In our efforts to protect ourselves and conform, we may come to believe things that do not accurately reflect who we are.

As we journey through life, it's crucial to pause and reflect, identifying beliefs that no longer benefit us. Signs of spiritual distress may manifest as a disconnection from our inherent qualities, leading to feelings of aimlessness, isolation, hopelessness, self-destructive language and behaviors, as well as fear, bitterness, and anger. Life's path encourages us to peel away any layers of conditioning, address the untruths, and embark on a journey of rediscovering ourselves.

Tracy found herself struggling to understand herself and the journey she was on. She was desperate to get to the root of her chronic illness and knew it was related to the disconnection from her true self and her place in the world. She shares with us how one of the ways she journeyed back was through a committed yoga practice.

For some of us, Eastern healing disciplines may fall outside our belief systems. If this is where you find yourself, we ask that you remain curious. In our efforts to learn about ancient breathing practices, we found that "breath" and "spirit" share the same origin in many languages. So, it's not inconceivable that practices like meditation, yoga, tai chi, and qi gong can lead us back to our true spirit.

Tracy's dedication to her personal growth and development is evident. Now a certified yoga instructor, she hopes to inspire others to embark on their own journeys toward self-discovery and inner peace.

"Like others before me, I was drawn to yoga in search of myself. I yearned for a practice that would not only strengthen my body but also quiet my mind and nourish my soul. Through overcoming obstacles, both mental and physical, yoga helped me to find a sense of belonging within myself and in the world around me.

It was evident in my early practice that I had lost my identity. I spent most of my life hiding behind a mask to cope with life's circumstances and had forgotten who I was. My mentor always says, "If there's emotional resistance in your body, yoga will find it." I struggled to hide deep sadness, anger, shame, and loneliness while portraying a happy, confident person to the outside world. I had a hard time loving and accepting myself, and every time I got close to success or happiness, I would self-sabotage. I persisted in my practice because something told me to trust the process. Just breathe.

On the mat, I allow my breath to guide my movements, working to find the right balance between physical effort and ease. I sink deeper into a pose as my breath allows, lightening up as my breath becomes heavy. The world fades away as I become completely immersed in my practice.

I discovered that power resides in stillness. I can witness thoughts coming and going without judgment or attachment. Irritations fade without the fuel of my attention. And instead of relenting when things get tough, I can pause in the discomfort and ask myself, What do I need? Is my foundation steady? Can I find ease with a simple lift of the heart? When I practice being present, non-reactive, and intentional on the mat, I am better able to carry those qualities off the mat and into my daily life.

Spiritual challenges happen off the mat. With a meditative discipline like yoga, I am able to cultivate a sense of calm and clarity that helps me navigate life's challenges. By staying present and non-reactive, I can approach difficult situations with a greater sense of awareness and understanding. This allows me to respond in a more intentional and thoughtful manner, rather than being driven by old wounds or external circumstances.

From a place of awareness, acceptance, compassion, forgiveness, and the knowing that I control my responses, life is immeasurably better. I feel connected again to that fun-loving spirit inside me. Yoga helps me live more intentionally, and as a result, I'm creating a much deeper and fuller life experience. Often, there is room for joy."

As we navigate life's obstacles, we have the opportunity to shed old beliefs and embrace our true selves, allowing us to become who we were always meant to be. By slowing down and connecting with ourselves, we can tap into our inner wisdom and find clarity and purpose. This enables us to make conscious choices that align with our values and bring us closer to living a meaningful and fulfilling life.

Finding spirituality in community.

Belonging goes to the essence of what we are; it addresses our humanity and existence. Being with and for others connects us to our purpose. Tracy's sister Leigh and her husband work in an industry that requires them to move often. Finding community and belonging in each new city is crucial for their happiness, mental and physical health, and longevity. A close-knit bond with their new neighbors meets their most recent cross-country move, and they feel blessed with an immediate sense of belonging and connection to their new community.

After a few months, Leigh's house burns down in a wildfire along with over a 1,000 neighboring homes, leaving them without identity or a sense of belonging. Leigh shares a story:

"There is a gravitational pull to visit and just 'be' in our burned neighborhood. Without trees to screen us, when my car pulls up to where our house once stood, the neighbors see us and pull in, too. So we meet for a visit, a hug, a cry, a laugh, and maybe even a cup of coffee! They understand, and it is a balm to the soul.

Military police protect the neighborhood around the clock, and accessing our lot is a process. Today is the last day we can enter with only our driver's licenses. They tell me to pick up a city-issued residential placard authorized by the Chief of Police to allow access to restricted areas for fire victims.

After I pick up my placards, I sit alone in my car in an empty parking lot and sob. The placard that dangles from my rearview mirror is my only connection to my old home and our way of life. It is now the symbol that we once belonged somewhere.

A tap on the window startles me, and to my amazement, a woman and her llama are staring at me, asking that I roll down the window. The woman says she couldn't help but notice I was 'sad' and she wonders if I'd like to meet her friend. So out the door, I go. I mean, it's not every day a llama comes knocking on your window. The handler says llamas are incredible service animals and can sense when people are distressed; I fit the bill!

The two of them are there to spread some llama love to our community members in need, which happened to be me in that parking lot in front of the placard distribution center that day. So she lets me hug that sweet animal and reassures me that we are not alone; we are all in this together. I mean, nothing says love quite like a llama, right!?

After a while, I thank the incredible duo for being there in my time of need. I express my appreciation for making me feel a part of and supported by this wonderful community. I still belong.

What did she say in response, you might ask? I kid you not. She smiled at me and said, 'No probllama!'"

"Laughter is good medicine for the soul. Our world is desperately in need of more medicine." —Jim Stovall

Leigh's story is heavy, and yet the levity of the llama keeps us smiling. It reminds us that laughter is, indeed, good medicine. Laughter has the potential to affect the quality of our lives significantly. Humor helps relieve tension, reassures people, and draws us together. So, how can you bring more laughter into your life?

Even now, a few years after the tragedy, Leigh's region continues to heal from the devastation, but the strength and determination of its residents are inspiring. The community at large continues to rally around its members with kindness and support, showing us the best of humanity.

Finding spirituality in nature.

We met to discuss launching our business, The Seven Dimensions of Wellness, at Helen's picturesque farmhouse. The three of us sat outside for hours under a magnificent oak tree, sharing our ideas and stories and deepening the conversation about what it means to be well. A chorus of chirping birds, the canopy of leaves, endless possibilities, and shared excitement created an embodied experience.

Taking a leap of faith into the unknown, Helen moved from New York City to an old historical farmhouse in Connecticut. While she wavered at the decision to leave her home state, Helen instinctively knew this beautiful property was where she would continue her journey. Although she wasn't sure what new adventures awaited her, Helen immediately felt the shift inside. She explains:

"I had this gift of time which allowed me to truly sit with myself. As I sat outside in my yard—taking in all the beauty surrounding me—I had an amazing experience. Looking at the trees on the property, it was as if I was seeing the world around me in an entirely different way. It was so peaceful and quiet. A feeling washed over me, and I very clearly felt a spiritual connection to my surroundings and a tremendous opening inside. I knew I was right where I was supposed to be. I found my sanctuary. Since that day, years ago, I have learned so much about my spiritual wellness. I understand my creative talents are gifts I am meant to share, and my challenging past led me to deepen my knowledge so I could counsel others on how we are each connected through our human experiences.

When I really need to ground myself, I sit under one of my trees and just be. I close my eyes, breathe, and feel my connection with nature."

Nature is the medicine the soul needs.

Finding spirituality in the vastness of the universe.

A science enthusiast from an early age, Diane's daughter Brittany describes her spirituality as a practice steeped in science. She speaks fondly of the night her dad woke her to witness a meteor shower in the middle of the night. They lay on the grass, looking into the universe, watching the magic unfold. While Brittany didn't understand it then, this was the moment she became one with the universe.

Deep in her soul, Brittany believes everything is interconnected. She shares that the tide needs the moon, mushrooms communicate through an impressive underground network of filaments called hyphae, the constellations are energies that mirror the energies within us, and intelligent life forms inhabit distant planets. We admit we can't hang on to the conversation when she turns to quantum theory and entanglement.

"If you want to find the secrets of the universe, think in terms of energy, frequency, and vibration." —Nikola Tesla

Today, Brittany feels she carries the energy of both her father and grandfather with her. She can feel her dad whenever she hears the Emerson, Lake & Palmer song "Lucky Man"; sometimes, she feels breathless, and other times, the visit is of great comfort. While typically Brittany has difficulty showing her emotions through tears, whenever a memory of her grandfather washes over her, she gets a tight feeling in her abdomen as healing tears fill her eyes.

It's easy to understand why Brittany became drawn to the vastness of the universe as a child, but when asked why her attraction deepened, she responds, *"I needed to feel small. To feel human. If you are small, your problems can't be that big."*

What is my purpose?

Our friend Patty shares a part of her journey of discovering her purpose and connecting with something greater than herself.

"When my husband died at 49, I had a Christian burial. I was never a go to church every Sunday person, but I attended semi-regularly over the years. The first service I attended after my husband died, I left partway through. I didn't find that it made me feel better to be there; I found it made me very sad. I was jealous of the people who had that faith, where anyone who died went to a better place. I wasn't there. How could God think a better place for my husband was away from his two boys?

Sometime over the last 15 years, since my husband passed away, I have come to find peace with my spirituality. I have taken the foundation of a Sunday ritual and tweaked it so that it works for me. I think my spirituality lives and breathes in me, not through some person standing in front of me telling me to believe only what they believe.

I am a caring person who believes you should always help others when you can. I found strength in volunteering to care for people at the end of their life journey. Something in me knows that I was meant to do this. Did a higher power lead me here, or did I find this because I was willing to be open to other forms of spirituality? Does it matter how I got here?"

On her journey, Patty found one of her gifts in the ability to comfort others at the end of their lives. She finds strength and purpose in volunteering for Hospice patients. According to many, like Patty, who assist the dying, people want to remember the kind deeds, connections, and love they experienced, not material possessions or accomplishments. Jack Kornfield, spiritual teacher and author of *A Path with Heart*, shares, "The things that matter most in our lives are not fantastic or grand. They are the moments when we touch one another and when we are there in the most caring way. This simple and profound intimacy is the love that we all long for."

"The meaning of life is to find your gift. The purpose of life is to give it away." —Pablo Picasso

The truth is, we don't need to be a famous painter or send a rocket ship into space to impact the world. Patty found one of her gifts in being of service to others. Underneath the circumstances, the pain, and the masks we wear, there is love. Love is the highest energetic vibration. Allowing love connects us to our light, our brilliance. In essence, love is fuel. What makes ordinary people extraordinary is using the love inside us to serve others.

If we let go of what we think spirituality should be and focus on what makes us feel connected to ourselves, our hearts, and others, we find its meaning. When we act out of kindness, compassion, and love, we align with our soul's purpose. Ultimately, we leave behind a legacy of love and connection with others. We need each other. This reminds us to sprinkle kindness everywhere.

Thinking back to the beginning of this chapter, "inner light" is the definition we like most to define spirit. Bringing awareness to ourselves and identifying what complexities in life dim our light allows us the choice to let those things go. Do you ever notice you have boundless energy when immersed in something you love? Finding what aligns deep within us is a source of that energy; it turns up our light.

If you need help figuring out where to start, find a practice to help quiet the mind, ground yourself in nature, do random acts of kindness, or find an organization you feel connected to and volunteer for them without expectation. You are like a million stars. Now, go light up the world. The universe is waiting for us to shine.

IT'S AN INSIDE JOB:
Practices for self-regulation

This loving-kindness, metta meditation, is adapted from a 2,500-year-old practice that teaches us to cultivate a love for ourselves in the same way we love others:

Find a comfortable place to sit, close your eyes, and breathe deeply. Bring to mind someone you love, someone you can easily show affection to, such as a child or a beloved pet. Imagine being in their company and experiencing in your body the natural warmth you have for their well-being and happiness. Send them your deepest gratitude:

May you be happy.
May you be loved.
May you be safe and protected.
May you find peace.

Allow each sentence to exude compassionate energy and love. After you've felt some natural gratitude for this loved one's well-being, expand this exercise to another person you care about. Recite the same basic sentences that communicate the aim of your heart. Gradually extend the meditation to additional family members and friends.

May you be happy.
May you be loved.
May you be safe and protected.
May you find peace.

When the sentiments of joy and love for others have become strong, turn back to include yourself. This may be challenging at first, but keep repeating these loving intentions despite any resistance or struggles that may emerge. Allow feelings of joy to slowly permeate your body and mind until you feel grounded in love.

May I be happy.
May I be loved.
May I be safe and protected.
May I find peace.

Now recite the same basic statements, adding neutral individuals, difficult people, and adversaries; keep expanding until you can experience compassion for everyone.

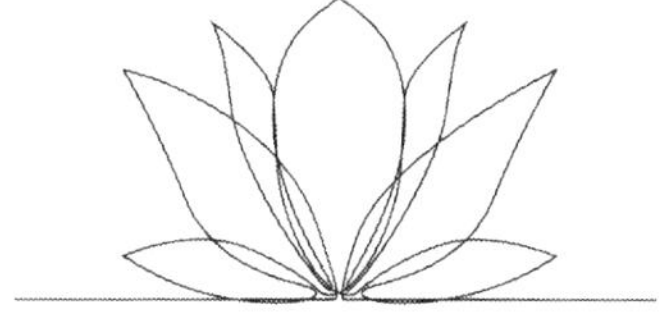

Physical

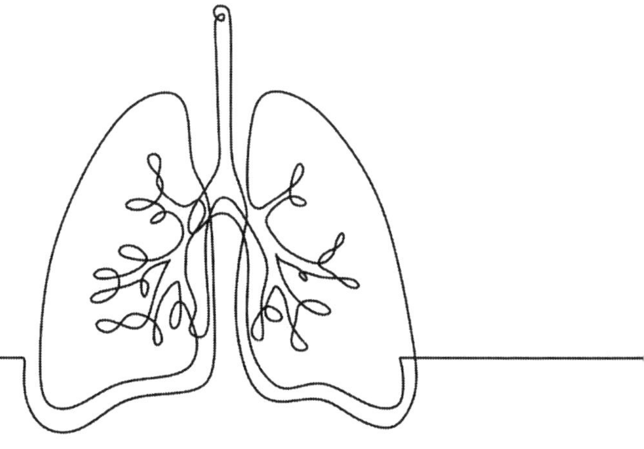

I am aware of
my body's brilliance
and tune into it
for messages.

“Listen to your body;
it always knows the right answer.”

—Kris Carr

Chapter 9

Physical Wellness

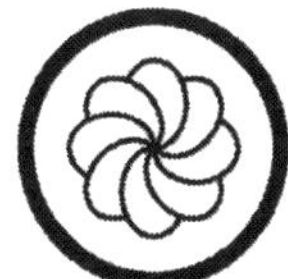

There is no greater cause for wonderment than the human body. It is capable of remarkable feats, adapting to different environments, and serving as a daily reminder of nature's beauty and complexity. Amidst our obsession with its outer appearance, the human body performs everyday miracles that often go unnoticed. Every moment of every day, our body tirelessly carries out countless functions that keep us alive and functioning.

We experience the world thanks to our senses, whether it's the taste of a fantastic meal, the feel of a warm embrace, the beauty of a sunset, or the sound of music. These sensory experiences connect us to the world and bring us joy, pleasure, and a deeper understanding of our surroundings. They remind us that life is meant to be experienced and enjoyed. Our bodies are the vessels through which we can fully immerse ourselves in the wonders of existence.

Physical wellness means listening to, nourishing, and caring for our body for optimal health and function.

Let's start with some incredible facts. Did you know the human body is constantly regenerating itself? It makes a new outer layer of skin every month and a new skeleton every ten years. In addition, our stomach lining renews every four to five days to prevent the stomach from literally digesting itself. Did you know that the number of bacteria in the body may be similar to the number of human cells? Imagine two to six pounds of bacteria inhabit the digestive tract of a human, and they play a crucial role in digestion, immunity, and even mental health.

The human body is alive with wonder. It is designed to protect and heal us and thrives when we give it the right things. Our body can be our most powerful guide if we take the time and effort to listen, understand, and care for it. When we shift our mindset to see our body as our most prized possession, we are more likely to fuel, condition, and care for it that way.

We are familiar with emotional intelligence (EQ) from Chapter 4, but another type of intelligence is just as critical to overall wellness: body intelligence (BQ). BQ focuses on being sharp and sensitive about what is happening inside. The body doesn't speak our language but it communicates through sensations, emotions, and physical cues. Body intelligence broadens our view by looking inside for answers; it makes us aware of the vast amount of knowledge stored in our cells. With a growth mindset, BQ helps us accept our emotions and inner experiences and encourages us to make conscious decisions in line with our true selves. We inspire others to connect with us authentically by becoming more deeply in touch with our truth and challenges.

Consider a time when you realized you were out of alignment; maybe you needed to leave a toxic job or end a relationship. What was happening in your body? Did you get a feeling that something was constantly tugging at you? Was there any intestinal distress? Was your back bothering you, or did you have an issue with your legs, knees, or feet? These are experiences we need to delve deeper into; they can often be signals from our body that something is not right and that we need to make a change.

"My body is a compass, and it does not lie."
—Terry Tempest Williams

Now, think about a moment when everything was going perfectly. Do you remember the feeling of being on the right track and energized by your choices? There is a sense of being in the flow of life, and the body says, "YES!" or "Thank you!" Imagine that resonance, like tuning into a radio station when your favorite song comes on. Deep contentment and harmony are what we are experiencing. These sensations signal we are on the right path and making choices in line with our true selves. These sensations may be our finest source of guidance.

We become more conscious by paying attention to and giving importance to our body's flashing lights. By acknowledging and honoring the signals our body sends us, we can tap into a deeper level of self-awareness. It allows us to recognize our emotions, physical sensations, and responses to different situations. This heightened consciousness will enable us to navigate life with greater clarity and alignment, ultimately leading to a more fulfilling and authentic existence. Recognizing the interplay between our physical and emotional states highlights the profound mind-body connection, emphasizing that our well-being is a holistic experience.

Body intelligence is the capacity to recognize, interpret, and respond to the data, signals, and sensations that the body sends us. This type of intelligence is also referred to as somatic intelligence or kinesthetic intelligence. Developing body intelligence requires practice and self-awareness, as well as a willingness to listen and trust the wisdom of our own bodies. These are some examples of body intelligence at work:

— Bringing attention to the health of our nervous system; the link between our mind and body.
— Recognizing that everything that affects the mind also impacts the body.
— Listening and responding to our body's signals.
— Bringing the same kindness to ourselves as we would a good friend.
— Focusing on what sustains us: real food, clean water, rest, movement, connection, love, and purpose.
— Asking questions and using our body's wisdom as a compass for making informed decisions.
— Valuing our intuition over any outside voice.
— Grounding ourselves and being present no matter where we are.

Listen, watch, and feel how our body responds to life.

To practice body intelligence, we begin our Monday meetings with Helen leading us through a body scan meditation—not a typical meeting icebreaker! We take the time to observe and sit with any sensations or feelings that arise without passing judgment. This practice helps us start the week with mindfulness and presence, allowing us to navigate challenges effectively. We learn to listen to our bodies and become more attuned to any signals they send us.

To start the exercise, Helen has us close our eyes, and we begin to connect with our breath. We move our awareness from the left foot to the right, the left and right legs, continuing to make our way to the top of the head, breathing deeply and opening our awareness to any sensations of pain, tension, discomfort, or ease.

One particular Monday, Tracy reported feeling tightness on her right side. After exploring the sensation further, she realizes she has been feeling stressed, "I feel this way whenever a chapter is in a state of muck. There is a sense of pressure, and I want to slow us down." The body communicates by sending signals of discomfort or ease, which can indicate underlying emotions or thoughts. By paying attention to these signals during a body scan, we can gain insight into our emotional well-being and address any areas of imbalance or stress. A sense of ease can also reaffirm that we are on the right track.

Tracy's awareness enabled us to discuss our process, validate each other, and return to a place of trust where our work eventually comes together. The body scan presents a unique opportunity to observe our sensations without judgment and gives us the space to ask into them. By identifying and understanding a source of tension, we can promote communication and reopen pathways for creativity and collaboration. This self-awareness allows us to see ourselves more clearly so we can cultivate a sense of trust in our abilities and intuition.

"The place where your greatest fears live is also the place where your greatest growth lies." —Robin Sharma

When we focus on our bodies, one of the first questions that comes to mind is, "Why are we so uncomfortable being uncomfortable?" As soon as we realize we are on the struggle bus, we want to get off at the first stop. This aversion to discomfort is deeply ingrained in our human nature. We are wired to seek pleasure and avoid pain, which often leads us to resist or avoid difficult situations. However, embracing discomfort can be a powerful catalyst for growth and personal development.

Our system is wired for safety. Being safe is necessary in certain situations, but constantly seeking comfort can hinder our ability to challenge ourselves and reach our full potential. We all seek ease in our familiar routines, and because of this, we risk getting trapped in our comfort zones. It may be that we eat at the same restaurants, take the same route to work, go to the same classes at the gym, and most of us socialize with the same groups of people—but if we never venture beyond the familiar and comfortable, we risk missing out on all that life has to offer.

Have you ever wanted to improve your diet? Exercise more often? Start a new career? Challenge your old belief system? Seek personal growth? Heal yourself? Guess what! All those changes require us to move outside our comfort zones through stages of difficulty. Learning to embrace discomfort as a necessary part of personal growth and development is pivotal. Making significant changes all at once, however, can feel unsafe to our nervous system, often sending us back to where we started. The key is taking small steps to increase that "safety zone."

Pain is talking; are you listening?

Discomfort is one of the most obvious ways the body communicates with us. Pain is a neurological function. It occurs when an alarm signal is activated, followed by the transmission of a pain message through our brain system. Pain is a flashing light informing us of issues with bodily function, when our mental health needs care, or when we are out of sync with our true selves.

Estimates suggest that 20% of the world's population suffers from chronic pain daily. Efforts to manage chronic pain and improve the quality of life for those affected by it typically involve medical treatments, pain management medicines, and physical therapy. Yet, despite a very advanced medical system, pain management is often prioritized over finding and fixing the mental, physical, and spiritual root causes. This emphasizes the need for a more holistic approach to pain treatment that targets the underlying causes at their root.

We are conditioned to suppress or hide our unease rather than allow it to fuel our curiosity for understanding. Pain is easily understood when associated with a physical event, such as a broken limb, an accident, or an overuse injury. Still, it becomes more challenging when no such event can be identified. When experiencing mental or emotional distress, it is common to automatically think things like "I shouldn't be feeling this way" or "How can I make this go away?" Avoiding uncomfortable feelings by refusing to acknowledge their existence is a losing strategy. This resistance may result in more of the very things we're attempting to ignore.

So what is all this talk about resistance? Simply put, resistance is the refusal to accept what is. We are here to feel so we can understand ourselves—mentally, physically, and spiritually. We can ask deeper into our discomfort by allowing and accepting what is. What element of reality are we fighting right now: ourselves, our emotions, another person, an event, or an experience? Any struggle (particularly one that repeats) asks us to be present, pay attention, be curious, and ask why. Mindfully sitting in discomfort can help inform us of any unfulfilled emotional or physical needs. When done with self-compassion, sitting with discomfort can be a constructive way to explore and address what needs tending to, leading to personal growth and enhanced well-being.

Inflammation is at the root of most diseases.

Inflammation is the body's response to cellular damage. Anything that puts the body in danger, such as infections, viruses, wounds, exposure to toxins, and even emotional stress, can trigger it. As a result of that defensive reaction, chemicals are produced that may excite nerve endings and cause pain. The pain is a warning signal that something is wrong in the body and needs some attention.

It is essential to tell the difference between short-term (acute) and long-term (chronic) inflammation because one may be beneficial, and the other might be harmful. Here is a recent exchange that took place between our good friend Jeff and Tracy:

Jeff: *"I'm confused. Is inflammation good or bad?"*

Tracy: *"Yes."*

Jeff: *"Wait, what?"*

Tracy: *"Ha! I mean, it's both. Inflammation is a defense response our immune system uses to free our body from infection, injury, or illness. That's good! This type of inflammation is called acute inflammation, and it goes away when the infection or damage to bone or tissue heals. Chronic inflammation, however, is like being in a dysregulated state. It is inflammation that doesn't turn itself off, so that's when it can become a problem."*

Joint pain, skin disorders (rashes, swelling, skin tags, and discoloration), headaches, insulin resistance, excessive mucus production, digestive issues, and fatigue are all potential indicators of chronic inflammation. Psst! Our body is talking to us! As a society, we are enmeshed in chronic conditions that are taxing our systems and keeping us ill as a result of our efforts to manage discomfort and normalize symptoms that are not normal. Symptoms are the body's messengers. If our only aim is to eliminate the symptom without finding the root cause, the body will find another way to alert us, just like the wolf that hides in the dark, waiting for us to falter so it can pounce and get the attention it craves. We hear so much about inflammation because chronic inflammation can lead to more severe conditions like Alzheimer's disease, cancer, inflammatory bowel disease, liver disease, rheumatoid arthritis, and type 2 diabetes when a root cause is not found.

Therefore, paying attention to our body's flashing lights and addressing underlying causes is important, rather than just treating the symptoms. A holistic approach to health can help prevent more severe conditions from developing due to chronic inflammation.

Learning to decode the symptoms.

In the Emotional Wellness chapter, we learned that when we resist emotions, we internalize them. Buried emotions may appear in various ways, causing physical sensations of distress or pain. The longer the pain persists, the more probable it is that it will become chronic and cause illness. Regardless if the underlying cause of pain is physical, psychological, or spiritual, our body holds the answers on how to decode the symptom.

Using BQ, let's connect to where emotions may settle in the body. "My boss is a pain in the neck," "I can't stomach this," and "I need to get this off my chest" are idioms reflecting how the body communicates where emotions settle. Many of us have difficulty naming emotions or understanding their relationship to our physical well-being; we grew up being told not to cry, "get over it," "be strong," or "there's no reason to be afraid." The underlying message is that having emotions is a negative experience. So, instead of allowing them, we repress them, and they get stuck.

According to Dr. Bradley Nelson, author of *The Emotion Code,* these trapped emotions can build up, causing pain, dysfunction, and disease. They can also impose a heavy mental and emotional toll, influencing how we think and behave, as well as our degree of success and prosperity. The most repressed emotions can gather around our hearts, making it hard to give and receive love. This can result in feelings of heaviness, tension, or physical discomfort.

We asked Diane to share a story about how her body spoke to her during a challenging time many years ago:

"I developed an open wound on the top of my right hand. It appeared as a small cut that began to spread, although I had no memory of injuring myself. Self-care wasn't a priority then, so it took a few weeks before I scheduled an appointment. I was annoyed when the doctor asked, 'What's going on in your life right now?' I didn't have time for small talk; I just wanted a solution to the problem. So, I gave my standard 'busy but good' reply.

He kept asking me probing questions, which just irritated me further. Finally, to stop the inquisition, I admitted I was going through a divorce and had three young kids. At that moment, he looked at me with very kind eyes and said, 'Your body is trying to tell you something; maybe your wound reflects your emotions. I will give you something so it's not receptive to infection, but your soul also needs care.' It was a light bulb moment for me."

We admire the doctor's insight, whole-body approach, and belief in the body's ability to heal. Instead of recommending medication to mitigate her stress, the doctor empowered Diane to ask herself what she needed during this time. Diane felt the "Yes" resonance in her body in response to the doctor's observations and chose to tell her sisters and a close friend about her stress.

"Sometimes the only way to carry a heavy burden is to share it with another." —Jim Butcher

We don't know the details of your complex ecosystem, and we are not trained physicians. Still, we have learned from personal healing journeys and our experience working with clients in a health crisis that making simple lifestyle changes can alter the condition of our environment and dramatically impact our overall health and well-being.

Remember, the body is designed to heal itself but it struggles to do so when dysregulated. There is no magic bullet or fast remedy. Slowing down and making adjustments to our lifestyle—learning to truly nourish ourselves—can help minimize chronic inflammation and restore equilibrium. But keep in mind our diet is more than what we eat. Everything we take in, including what we watch, listen to (including our thoughts!), and surround ourselves with, can be either nourishing or stressful.

Empowerment is in our ability to choose. So, let's bring more awareness to nourishing ourselves and how it affects our physical, emotional, and spiritual wellness. Ultimately, caring for ourselves holistically can lead to a more balanced and harmonious state of being.

Want to flourish? You need to nourish.

The human body is like the best sports car in the world: a well-tuned machine. A sports car is a complex system with many parts that work together to do different jobs, just like the human body. Imagine the engine as the heart, the vehicle bus as the nervous system, and the electronic control units as the organs. The brain is the software. Add the high-tech safety sensors that tell us when something is wrong, and we can imagine ourselves as a shiny Ferrari!

When we own a Ferrari, we do everything we can to keep it in the best shape possible. It's likely to be the love of our lives. When we think of "nourishment," we think of premium fuel. Of course, this is a must for our Ferrari, but proper treatment for the vehicle includes care and maintenance for the entire system. In the same way, nourishment for our being is also multidimensional. When we use Body Intelligence, we are constantly reevaluating our relationship to how we are taking care of ourselves:

— Am I regularly feeding myself good thoughts?

— What is my relationship to alcohol, drugs, nicotine, caffeine, and junk food? How do they serve me?

— Are my relationships nourishing?

— How heavy is my toxic load?
— Is my work in line with my moral compass?
— Am I putting out the same kind of energy I wish to attract?
— How do certain foods make me feel?

During our years in the wellness industry, the most commonly asked question was, "What should I eat for better health?" We don't have all the answers—but the good news is our body does! Practicing body intelligence and tuning into our body will be our best guide toward a lifestyle that allows us to thrive.

If that's different from what you were hoping for in this chapter, the most straightforward answer we have is:

Eat real food! Avoid ultra-processed food products and use real food ingredients to create meals. A Mediterranean diet is a good example of an anti-inflammatory diet, but remember, real food is not limited to any specific diet or cuisine. Incorporating a wide variety of vegetables, fruits, whole grains, lean proteins, and healthy fats into your meals can provide essential nutrients and help reduce inflammation in the body. Don't forget the leafy greens.

Don't drink your calories! Eliminate sugary and chemically filled drinks.

Strive to consume the best quality foods available—organic and local are best.

Limit or avoid sugar and alcohol—moderation is essential when it comes to sugar and alcohol. However, avoiding these substances completely may benefit those with health concerns or who want healthier lifestyles.

Make sure you get enough protein, choose complex carbs from nature (like vegetables and fruit), and choose healthy fats. These are the building blocks for a healthy diet.

These five suggestions may provide outstanding mental and physical outcomes on their own. It doesn't take long to realize the advantages of making a few simple modifications—we recognize simple doesn't always mean easy!

The Environmental Wellness chapter discussed how homemade dishes with living food ingredients are the most nourishing and health-sustaining for all. If you need a visual of a "living" food, cut the bottom off a bunch of celery, place it on your windowsill in a shallow dish of water, and watch it grow. Or plant a garlic clove in the fall and watch it come up in late spring. The body receives the living energy it needs from these natural ingredients rich in vitamins, minerals, enzymes, and amino acids.

But we get it; preparing meals from scratch can initially seem time-consuming, expensive, and downright overwhelming. According to Dr. Eli Jarrouge, most metabolic health benefits come from what you STOP eating. Many of us are aware of the unhealthy foods we are consuming that are detrimental to our health. It's up to us to be radically honest and take responsibility for how we're nourishing ourselves. Would we put sludge in the engine of our Ferrari?

Try not to let the need for change stress you out; worrying too much about what, when, and how much to eat can also lead to inaction. Instead, start slow and make incremental changes. Remember, food labels are our first line of defense. Avoid the product when ingredients on a label are hard to identify. It isn't food. Real food rarely needs an ingredient label. Studies show that ultra-processed foods are highly inflammatory and can be linked to early death, full stop. So, start to phase them out.

Do you suffer from digestive discomfort or acne? Try an experiment where you remove inflammatory foods like sugar, gluten, and dairy from your diet for three weeks and notice any changes. Then, reintroduce them separately and be aware of your body's response. The mindset that you're experimenting out of love for your body can make the time and effort more operable. You're worth it!

Keep calm and eat with intention.

BQ reminds us that HOW we eat is as important as what we eat. Many of us eat our meals on the go, in front of the TV, or while scrolling on our phones. If we eat when stressed, distracted, or "dining on the dashboard," we do not allow our digestive systems to digest, absorb, and assimilate nutrients properly. Optimal digestion happens in a parasympathetic or relaxed state (it's called "rest and digest" for a reason!), where we are setting ourselves up to get the most benefit from the nutrients in our food. Mindful eating means pausing, expressing gratitude, and finding joy in the experience of nourishing ourselves. Creating rituals around meals can positively affect our physical health. Take a moment to sit and take in the beauty of the food. Your body will thank you for it!

You're a human being, not a human doing.

While daily movement and maintaining muscle mass are imperative for optimum health and longevity, listening to our body when it calls for rest is critical. We get it wrong when we think of rest as a reward for hard work when, in fact, rest should be prioritized to enhance productivity (as well as health and happiness!). Rest is one of the most underappreciated forms of nourishment; rest is foundational for wellness.

We live in a culture where exhaustion is a badge of honor, and "doing nothing" is seen as a lost opportunity. However, what is happening autonomously in the body while resting is profoundly important. Studies show that rest improves cardiovascular health and reduces blood pressure and cortisol levels. So it's not surprising to learn that women who don't take vacations have a higher occurrence of depression and, according to one report, a 50% higher risk of a heart attack.

"Almost everything will work again if you unplug it for a few minutes—including you." —Anne Lamott

We don't need research to tell us that resting is sometimes the most productive thing we can do. But if we've been living in a hurry for years, our nervous system may view slowing down as unsafe. Remember, if it's unfamiliar, the body may see it as a threat, even when it's beneficial. Notice if you feel resistance to resting. It may seem silly initially, but if you need practice, set the alarm for midday and unplug for 10 minutes. Give yourself permission to do absolutely nothing but close your eyes and breathe. As you increase the time spent at rest, you will rewire your brain to understand that stillness is not threatening.

Just breathe.

What do you do between 12 and 20 times a minute and 17,000 to 30,000 times a day, and you probably don't even realize you're doing it? We are saving one of the best forms of nourishment for last. Nothing is more important to our health and well-being than breathing. It may come as a surprise to learn that, as a species, humans have lost the ability to breathe correctly, with severe consequences. Journalist James Nestor, the author of the eye-opening book *Breath,* travels the world to figure out what went wrong and how to fix it.

According to Nestor's findings, most humans today breathe short, shallow breaths from their mouths without awareness. Unfortunately, we are missing out on the depth of this lifeforce energy and alerting our nervous system that danger is lurking. In addition, mouth breathing causes stress hormones to be released, keeping us in a constant state of fight or flight.

In response, the body turns on flashing lights to indicate that our breathing is causing damage, such as stress, anxiety, brain fog, high blood pressure, snoring, and, according to Dr. Mark Burhenne, from the podcast *Ask the Dentist* with Dr. Mark Burhenne, even cavities, and crooked teeth. Unfortunately, we don't know how to connect the symptoms to the underlying cause, and we risk creating more significant dysfunction and disease in our systems over time. Breathing in and out through the nose slows breathing and signals calm to the body.

Modern research shows that even minor changes in inhaling and exhaling can improve athletic performance, rejuvenate internal organs, stop snoring, asthma, and autoimmune diseases, and even straighten scoliotic spines. Even though none of this appears to be possible, it is.

One way to bring awareness to proper breathing is to curl up beside a dog at rest. Put your hand on its belly and feel the deep, rhythmic breathing that fills the entire body cavity as the dog breathes in and out through the nose. Move your hand to the chest, and you'll feel nothing. When a dog is stressed, however, they pant from the chest through the mouth.

Bringing consciousness to our breath through meditation, yoga, tai chi, and qi gong, which connect the mind, body, and spirit, can promote healing in the body. Furthermore, by practicing daily multidimensional self-care, we can tune in to our body's innate wisdom. Making self-care a habit is essential, so it becomes a natural reaction in challenging times.

Growing forward.

Listen to your body. Nourish your body. Challenge your body. Believe in your body. And most of all, love your body. It's the only one you have.

Wellness today necessitates personal accountability; we must advocate for ourselves in our fragmented healthcare system. Consider this: we go to a neurologist who knows the brain and only discuss our neurological issues. Then, we go to a cardiologist who specializes in the heart, and we only share information that we believe is relevant to them. We see a gastroenterologist who specializes in the digestive system to talk about our digestive issues. Who is connecting the dots and looking at the interplay between different systems in our body?

As we need treatment or guidance, it is wise to seek out a holistically-minded physician interested in the interconnectedness of our systems. It is our responsibility to act as wellness ecologists and be active participants in our healthcare decisions. We must strive toward health and never stop asking why. Learning our body's language, trusting it, and making proactive efforts to preserve and care for it can help us reach a higher level of well-being.

Recent findings show that only a fraction of our health issues are genetic. We give up control when we believe that our genes determine our future. Instead, our habits, practices, routines, eating patterns, and beliefs significantly impact our health and well-being. The good news is all of these things are in our control! It's time to switch from symptom management to a functional lens, where we look for the underlying causes.

Remember, our body can be our best friend and guide. It works to keep us healthy and safe and constantly gives us feedback about what it needs to thrive. By tuning in to its messages, we can take charge of our health, make changes for the better, and shape a brighter future. Let's start tuning in, embracing this powerful awareness, and nurturing our bodies for life.

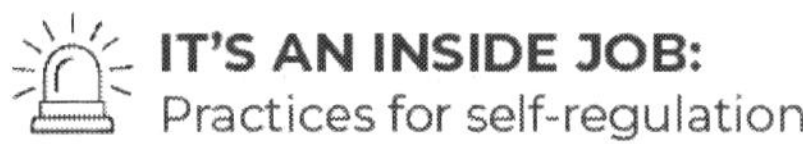

Dashboard warning lights and indicators alert us when we need to refill the washer fluid or check the engine; the body communicates with us similarly through sensations alerting us that something needs attention. BQ encourages us to be curious about how the body speaks so we can begin to understand its language. Ask your body questions like you would a close friend. Rather than ignoring or attempting to turn signals off, we can learn to befriend them as we practice interpreting their meaning.

Examples of self-examination: Is my stomach upset because of something I ate, or is it because I'm traveling this week, and travel always gives me a little anxiety? Is my shoulder stiff because I overexerted myself physically, or am I carrying too heavy of a burden? Is this headache attempting to gain my attention by suddenly appearing? What was happening in my life when this symptom first appeared? Is this symptom helping me to avoid something? Amy Scher, author of How to Heal Yourself When No One Else Can, offers a few common metaphors to consider when symptoms arise in certain body parts.

Back: Patterns of carrying everything, being unable to stand up for yourself, being stabbed in the back, being afraid to turn your back, turning your back on someone (guilt), living in the past, wishing you could go back and change something, having no backbone with others.
Legs/Knees/Feet: Fear of moving forward, being ungrounded, unsure of your next step, carrying too much emotional weight, and feeling stuck.
Shoulders: Carrying the weight of others, shouldering a burden or worry, giving or being given the cold shoulder, or trying to shrug something off to avoid conflict. Shoulders can also be linked to feeling pushed around.

Skin: Your skin acts as a barrier between you and the world. When symptoms show up on the skin, they may be linked to feeling like someone is getting under your skin, feeling unprotected against something, or feeling that you are itching or burning to release something.
Stomach/Intestines: Related to being unable to "digest" an experience, being sick with worry/guilt/fear, feeling disgusted or upset about something, feeling stuck or unable to let go of the old (constipation), or releasing unfelt terror (diarrhea).

Healing and Strengthening the Vagus Nerve

A health journey often feels like a complicated puzzle! We frequently overlook that the nervous system plays a role in developing chronic symptoms; therefore, healing and strengthening the vagus nerve may be a crucial component we're missing. Keep in mind that the nervous system is what connects the mind and body, making them one. A dysregulated nervous system can lead to a dysregulated body. Try incorporating some of these into your routine for toning the vagus nerve:

Cold Showers	Morning sunlight	Massage
Humming	Rest	Acupuncture
Singing	Laughing	Plant medicine
Chanting	Adaptogenic herbs	EFT-Tapping
Grounding	Gratitude	Hydration
Gargling	Breath work	Nature's wonder

Tending to Your Garden

Flowers need the right amount of water, sunlight, and nutrients to grow and flourish. Similarly, nutrition and lifestyle choices support or harm our inner garden, the gut microbiome.

Nourishing and healing our inner garden can be a critical missing piece to our health and well-being. Our guts are home to trillions of bacteria and microbes that inhabit the intestines and form the gut microbiota. Keeping this system balanced and happy is one of the keys to good health.

Signs your microbiome is out of balance:
— Sugar cravings
— Mood issues
— Digestive upset
— Chronic illness
— Skin rashes

Ways to support and heal your gut:
— Focus on macronutrients: protein, carbohydrates, and healthy fat.
— Eat the colors of the rainbow (think veggies!).
— Get plenty of fiber from high-nutrient whole foods.
— Enjoy fermented foods: yogurt, kefir, tempeh, miso, kimchi, sauerkraut.
— Limit sugar, decrease toxins, exercise + maintain a healthy weight.

Being curious about how we function can be beneficial to our overall well-being. Take in your role as a host to trillions of bugs with awe and wonderment, and tend to your inner garden by making decisions that prioritize the health and happiness of your gut microbiome.

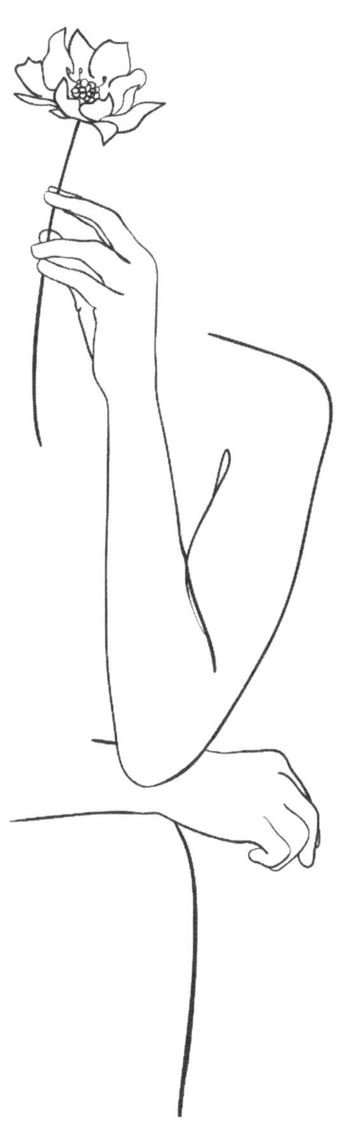

"Self-knowledge is medicine. Energy is medicine. Connection is medicine. Nature is medicine. Purpose is medicine. Food is medicine. Love is medicine."

—Helen Barnard

Chapter 10

A Path Forward

Peace, happiness, and good health are our responsibilities, and we must be relentless in our pursuit of them. It's an inside job. The first step in making positive changes in our lives is to raise our level of self-awareness. Then, with safety and support, we can muster the courage to be vulnerable and face the uncomfortable truths that may arise in our self-explorations. Accepting ourselves in our entirety and learning to bring love and compassion to those uncomfortable places alters everything in and around us. Accepting the past as part of the fabric of our being allows us the choice to create a beautiful path forward.

By breaking down the countless complexities of being human and focusing on seven key dimensions, we can see how everything we touch or are touched by affects our wellness in some capacity. Understanding the interconnectedness of these—physical, mental, emotional, social, environmental, spiritual, and intellectual—facets can help us make informed decisions that promote a more balanced and fulfilling life. Furthermore, recognizing that the wellness continuum is constantly changing emphasizes the importance of ongoing self-reflection, adaptation, and a holistic approach to health and wellness.

A key insight into the Seven Dimensions is that they are dynamic and interconnected. Changes in one dimension can influence others. For example, lowering stress levels (emotional) can positively impact physical wellness. Similarly, finding fulfillment in a job (occupational) can affect relationships outside of work (social).

The journey begins with an awareness of the body as a guide. By tuning into our sensations, we can tap into the wisdom within us. This awareness helps us make informed choices about our health and well-being. It allows us to identify areas that may need improvement and take proactive steps towards achieving balance and harmony in our lives.

We can witness how the body responds to different situations and experiences by bringing consciousness to our nervous system. This awareness allows us to behave in ways that align with our goals rather than react. Our ability to choose our response is our superpower. Developing a heightened sensitivity also enables us to recognize and work to release any stored tension or trauma, allowing for healing and growth on a deeper level. Ultimately, by honoring the wisdom of our bodies, we can create an enlightened path forward that reflects our true essence.

The past is in your head; the future is in your hands.

What is the path forward? We can do the work to understand ourselves better, but we won't see a clear path ahead until we define what's important to us. Take some time to determine what matters to you most. What are your ideals, and how do you want to make a difference? Once we have clarity on our values and goals, we can align our actions and decisions with them, creating a sense of purpose and direction. The journey ahead will be unique to each of us. As we change and grow, being on a path forward involves continuously reassessing and realigning with our true selves, allowing us to live a fulfilling and meaningful existence. Life is calling us to live on purpose.

For example, someone defines that family is the most important thing right now and wants a better work-life balance. They decide to prioritize spending quality time at home over working long hours. As a result, they adjust their schedule, delegate tasks, and set boundaries at work to ensure they have dedicated time for family. This alignment with their values brings them a sense of satisfaction and fulfillment as they can nurture relationships and create lasting memories with their loved ones.

The ability to shape our future is fundamental to our growth as human beings. This sense of control enables us to make choices, create goals, and act consistently with our ideals and objectives. A belief in our abilities gives us the confidence to take charge of our lives and make positive changes.

While the example above portrays creating a work-life balance as easily attainable, taking charge of life is rarely easy. The ability to directly influence and change our immediate environment to solve a problem or overcome adversity is known as primary control. It involves taking proactive steps and making choices that directly impact our circumstances. By taking charge, we can let go of the things that are undesirable or no longer serving us and add something that may improve our circumstances. This sense of agency fosters resilience and a belief in our capabilities, leading to increased satisfaction and well-being.

When we don't have control of our surroundings, we need a different approach to dealing with our challenges. Control becomes adapting and adjusting one's thoughts, attitudes, and emotions to overcome the situation. This is called secondary control. In the Environmental chapter, we shared an example of secondary control where Louie Zamperini, Victor Frankl, and Nelson Mandela chose to cultivate a sense of self-efficacy and resilience in the face of extreme adversity.

This type of agency focuses on accepting, finding meaning, and maintaining personal control even when circumstances cannot be changed. This allows us to navigate challenges with resolve and optimism, but developing this mindset requires practice and effort. It requires a shift in perspective and a willingness to let go of the need for control over external factors. By focusing on what we can control—our thoughts, attitudes, and behaviors —we can cultivate a sense of inner strength and empowerment that helps us navigate adversity with grace and resilience.

When we let go of the need to control external factors, we relieve ourselves of the burden of constantly trying to change our circumstances. Otherwise, we risk becoming mired in a cycle of negativity and frustration while perpetually feeling powerless over external factors. Instead, we can accept what is and focus on cultivating a positive mindset and finding solutions within ourselves. This shift in awareness and perspective empowers us to better approach challenges, knowing we can adapt and grow. We can't pretend it's easy, but we can work on building the self-assurance and stability necessary to weather life's inevitable storms.

Gratitude is an effective way to practice accepting what is and cultivating a positive mindset regardless of our challenges. By expressing gratitude for the things we have in our lives each day or looking for the positive in any situation, we train our minds to focus on the positive aspects rather than dwelling on the negatives. This helps us maintain a positive outlook and find solutions to adversity. Additionally, incorporating mindfulness techniques such as meditation or deep breathing exercises can help us stay present and approach challenges with a clear mind and open heart.

We lay the foundation for overall well-being when we see ourselves holistically and focus on self-care. Just like the farmer who works to ensure success by focusing on all the interconnected components of the farm, we must consider all of our interrelated dimensions and physical systems. Moreover, we must make connections to understand how our choices and habits affect us. Recognizing the interdependence of the seven dimensions can guide us toward choices that lead to a happier, healthier, and more satisfying existence.

— Intellectual: By having the power to choose, we create our lives.

— Emotional: There are no good or bad emotions. Waves of positive and negative energy flow through us, guiding our reactions to the world in and around us.

— Social: How we feel about ourselves affects every other relationship. We teach others to love us the way we love ourselves. Bringing compassion to ourselves at every age is critical to acceptance and self-love.

— Environmental: We can't always grow where we are planted; sometimes, we must change the environment. Our daily choices have a profound effect on our well-being.

— Occupational: Prioritizing balance and staying true to our values can increase personal fulfillment and job satisfaction. Balance requires deliberate effort to slow down and work at the rhythm of our nervous system. Overworking ourselves can cause us to ignore our biological needs.

— Spiritual: Our light shines brightly when we feel connected to ourselves, others, and our surroundings. It is our purpose to find our gifts and share them with others.

— Physical: The body is a brilliant tool for living; it is designed to keep us safe and heal itself. It can be our best guide If we take the time to understand and nourish it.

The path forward is to see yourself as the architect of your life. You have the power to choose your thoughts and responses, what you put into and onto your body, who you surround yourself with, and what you do with your time. Only you are aware of all the complexities of your ecological system, making YOU the most qualified expert on you. Learn to trust yourself. Life is beckoning you to live more deliberately and authentically.

Take responsibility for your one precious life and make intentional choices that align with the future you wish to create. It's an inside job.

Honor your journey.

IT'S AN INSIDE JOB:
Practices for self-regulation

When beginning a new practice or journey, particularly one aimed at enhancing well-being, it is essential to be conscious of where you are as a starting point and define what you seek. This awareness acts as a baseline assessment, offering insights about your behaviors, ideas, and general state to help keep you focused on your desired outcomes.

Remember that our state of being constantly changes as we evolve and respond to new situations. This emphasizes the importance of ongoing self-reflection, adaptation, and growth.

Summarize or rate where you are in each dimension, and clearly define where you want to be. Then, check in with yourself regularly, "Do my current thoughts and behaviors align with my values and goals?" This self-reflection allows us to make necessary adjustments and empowers us to actively shape our future.

My Seven Dimensions:

— Intellectual Wellness:

— Emotional Wellness:

— Social Wellness:

— Environmental Wellness:

— Occupational Wellness:

— Spiritual Wellness:

— Physical Wellness:

Personalize this exercise to fit your needs and preferences. Use our definitions or define them for yourself. You can journal your thoughts and progress or seek support from a coach, mentor, or accountability partner.

Rediscover Yourself

Explore who you are in a new light. Be courageous and vulnerable. Be radically honest with yourself. Take some time to ponder these questions and notice the patterns and themes that emerge.

— When do I most feel alive?

— What brings me joy?

— What brought me joy as a child?

— What are my strengths?

— What do I want my legacy to be?

Notice any common threads or recurring interests that arise from your explorations. Pay attention to the activities or experiences that consistently bring you fulfillment and joy. Trust in your unique qualities and let them shine through as you navigate your journey. Embrace the things that brought you joy as a child, as they often hold clues to your strengths and passions. By understanding and leveraging your strengths, you can positively impact others and create a legacy that is authentic to you.

Allow these reflections to guide you toward aligning your purpose with your thoughts and actions. Remember, it's never too late to align your passions with your future and leave a lasting mark on the world.

You've got this! Enjoy your adventure!

Epilogue

At the end of many journeys, where we arrive is not where we expected; this is the case for the three of us. We launched this project to inspire a broader sense of self-awareness as a means to better health. By breaking down the countless complexities of being human and focusing on seven key facets, we can see how everything we touch or are touched by affects our wellness in some capacity.

While this is still true, what we gained along the way is an even greater understanding of how much richer our lives are when we are unapologetically authentic, kind, and willing to grow. Sharing our experiences and conveying information we learned through our education and hardships allowed us to bring even more consciousness into our lives throughout the creative process; we were essentially living the book along the way.

The safety and support we gifted each other gave us the courage to be vulnerable and face some uncomfortable truths. When we learn to love and accept all of ourselves, including the parts we find most challenging, our entire world shifts. What continues to be reaffirmed for us is that peace, happiness, and good health are our responsibilities, and we are each unique in how we pursue them. Holding space for one another, holding each other accountable, and loving each other are essential components of our journey forward.

Our quest for a deeper understanding of ourselves and of the world around us doesn't end with this book. It's another new beginning. We hope the same is true for you.

"Sharing stories can help ease the burden of others, spark curiosity, and express the power of connectivity."

—Diane Hubbard

Chapter 12

Continuing the Conversation

Book clubs provide an opportunity for social interaction and engagement with like-minded individuals who share a love of reading. Sharing our stories and experiences in a safe and supportive environment can be a powerful way to ease emotional burdens and promote healing. Book club members often have diverse backgrounds, experiences, and viewpoints. This variety of perspectives and experiences enhances the conversation and promotes deeper mutual understanding.

While sharing stories at book club may be therapeutic for some, it is important to note that it is not always the best option for everyone. Some individuals may prefer to process their experiences privately or through professional therapy. We hope you will follow your instincts and continue the conversation in a way that is right for you.

Chapter Two: Seven Dimensions

A healthy nervous system pendulates back and forth, moving fluidly between states, creating rhythm, balance, and harmony for all the functions of our body. Knowing these responses can help us gain insight into what makes us do what we do and allow us to live more consciously.

1. Does knowing that your body prioritizes safety over everything change how you see your instincts and responses? Does seeing

yourself as a system allow you to "accept and work with your body's natural tendencies rather than feel something's wrong with you?

2. What settings or relationships give you a sense of security and make you feel "at home"?

3. Before reading this book, did you see yourself through a multidimensional lens?

4. Would you add another element to the seven dimensions?

Chapter Three: Intellectual

Intellectual wellness is being curious, open to differing views, and willing to challenge everything you think you know. It also means being aware of our power to create.

Balance in this dimension is about being open to exploring new topics and challenging everything you think you know. It is about being ever curious and aware of our power to create.

1. You can live by design or default; which best describes you?

2. Do you consider yourself a lifelong learner?

3. Were you able to identify any subconscious beliefs from your childhood that you hold onto but no longer serve you?

4. In what ways are you creative? Do you see yourself as the creator of your life?

5. The mind replays what the heart wants to heal. Do you pay atten-

tion to your patterns?

Chapter Four: Emotional

Emotional wellness is understanding ourselves and embracing life's challenges. It is acknowledging, accepting, and sharing feelings of anger, fear, sadness, distress, hope, love, joy, and happiness in a productive manner

Emotions are bodily sensations triggered by external or internal stimuli; they play a crucial role in our lives and can influence our behaviors, thoughts, and decision-making processes. The most empowering realization is that, with conscious awareness, we can choose how we respond.

1. Do you see emotions as good and bad? How do your emotions shape your reactions to the world around you?

2. Children often lack the vocabulary and understanding to express and make sense of their feelings. Can you identify unresolved childhood emotions that may continue to impact you as an adult?

3. The more you can sit with uncomfortable sensations, the faster the discomfort disappears; this highlights the importance of facing challenges head-on instead of avoiding them. Are you willing to sit on the struggle bus, or do you want off at the first stop?

4. Do you regularly practice acceptance and self-love? If yes, how? If, not, why not?

Chapter Five: Social

Social wellness is establishing and nurturing positive relationships with self, family, friends, and co-workers while maintaining healthy boundaries. It is realizing that every relationship we have is directly impacted by how we feel about ourselves.

How we feel about ourselves directly affects every other relationship. To maintain authentic connections, we must nourish ourselves and others with love, compassion, and empathy.

1. If you were to list your most important relationships, would YOU top your list?

2. Can you see connections between your earliest bonds with your caregivers and your relationship patterns as an adult?

3. Do you surround yourself with others who embody the vibration of who you want to be?

4. A judgmental lens is a messenger to find inner healing. Are you aware of your critical thoughts (about yourself and others) and how they can hinder relationships?

Chapter Six: Environmental

Environmental wellness is being in tune with how our everyday life impacts us and taking responsibility for what we're exposed to in our homes, work, relationships, and greater surroundings. It is

being aware of how our environment affects us and, in turn, how we affect the environment.

Environmental wellness is taking responsibility for what we are exposed to in our homes, work, relationships, and greater surroundings. We can improve our lives by changing our environment—thoughts, habits, surroundings, nourishment, and relationships.

1. Does seeing your body as a precious vehicle for living encourage you to nourish yourself differently?

2. Can you see how your life mirrors your internal world?

3. The body has a limited capacity to detoxify. Do you pay attention to your toxic load?

4. Can you identify things in your environment that negatively impact your health or hinder your growth? Is altering them in your control? If you answered yes, what is holding you back?

Chapter Seven: Occupational

Occupational wellness is gaining personal fulfillment from a job, career, or volunteer position while still maintaining balance in life.

Being healthy at work means being true to ourselves, standing up for what we believe in, establishing healthy boundaries, and finding fulfillment in what we do.

1. How did the messages you received about work as a child impact your current view of earning an income?

2. Do you work for "You, Inc.” or someone else?

3. Is your work fulfilling or a means to an end?

4. Is your work in line with your values?

Chapter Eight: Spiritual

Spiritual wellness is our deepest level of consciousness. It is the state of being connected to something greater than ourselves while finding meaning and purpose in life.

Spirituality is a universal language that allows us to feel a sense of belonging and connect with something greater than ourselves. Connecting deeply with ourselves and others while doing what we love has a powerful magnetic vibration. Everything we need will be in alignment with that energy.

1. Do you connect to an inner knowing? Do you know your purpose?
2. What makes you feel most alive? Do you notice that when you're doing something you love, you essentially "turn your light on"
3. Do you connect to the notion that your true essence, or your spirit, is the witness/listener of your thoughts?
4. In what circumstances do you feel most genuine? Can you embrace the positive and negative aspects of your being and show up as your complete self?

Chapter Nine: Physical

Physical wellness means listening to, nourishing, and caring for our body for optimal health and function.

The body is a wonderland, capable of remarkable feats and adapting to various conditions. Body intelligence is essential for personal growth and takes time and practice.

1. Do you pay attention to your body's flashing lights? Are you most interested in turning them off, or do you search for a root cause?

2. The body thrives on natural ingredients rich in vitamins, minerals, enzymes, and amino acids. Do you prioritize "living foods?"

3. Do you see rest as a reward for hard work or an underrated form of nourishment?

4. When we use body intelligence, we regularly re-evaluate how we care for ourselves. Do you continually reevaluate potentially harmful habits? Substances? Social media? Shopping? Junk food? How are they serving you?

5. What nourishment can you add to your life to improve your well-being?

Chapter Ten: A Path Forward

We must trust our body as a guide and make conscious decisions that align with our values and goals to design a life that brings joy, fulfillment, and well-being. Personal growth comes through introspection, deliberate thought, and action.

1. Do you see yourself differently after reading this book, if yes, how?

2. What is your biggest takeaway?

3. How will you continue to create your desired life?

Unsung Heroes

We acknowledge that our parents and siblings served as our greatest teachers. We value the lessons they instilled in us and their impact on our personal development. They will forever be a part of the tapestry of our lives.

In no particular order, a heartfelt thanks to those who championed the creation of this book: The Arnold Family, Jeff L. Hubbard, Nick, Brittany, Bethany, Stallone, Melissa, Karen Rubenstein, Patty Murphy, Dan Leven, Jill Teas, Leigh Pierini, Dr. John Chandler, Nicole Reilly, Scott Sweeney, Dean Markadakis, Cheryl Della Pietra, Carrie Patterson, Deb Dormody, Dr. Shannon Forshey, Amanda Soucier, Cherise Colombo, Sage Brody, Carol Pierini, Deb Davis, Kim Mathieu, Rose Mihaly, Valerie Taylor, Tammy Snee and Lorna Davis.

A special thanks to Sarah Leathers, CEO of Healing Meals Community Project, for bringing us together and sharing her wisdom.

Thanks to The Marshall Fire Community for helping us locate the sweet alpaca and his handler, Patti Fisher of FishFam Alpacas. Patti is a testament to the power of community. She reminds us that we can all make a difference in someone's life by offering kindness and compassion.

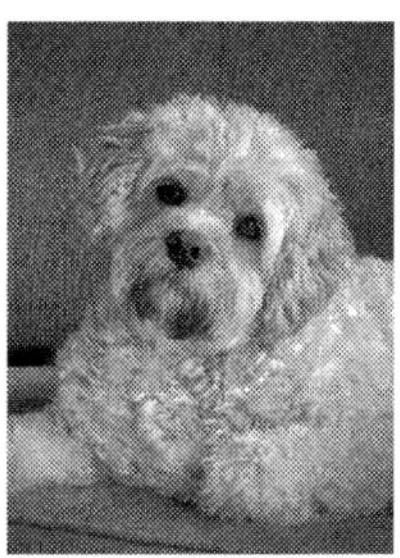

Leo the dog, our furriest friend and staunch supporter.

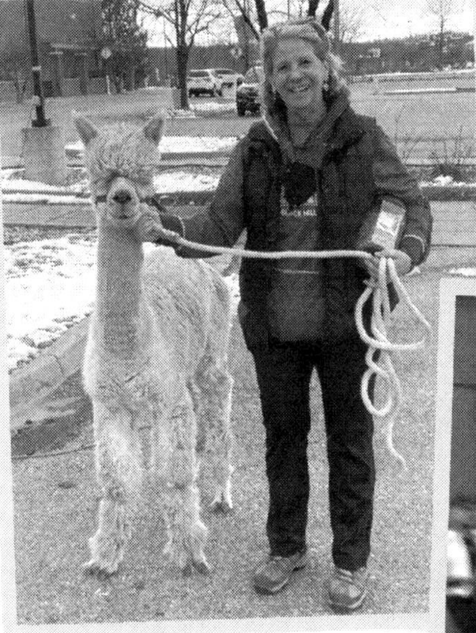

"No Probllama"

Tracy's sunny
exterior on the go.

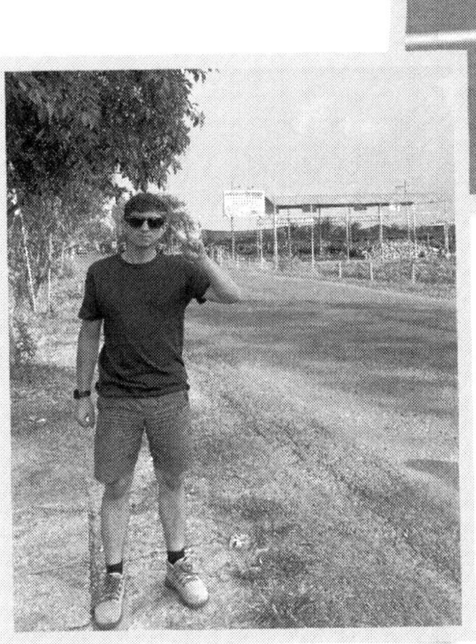

Nick in Vietnam.

Chapter 14

For a Better Understanding

Reading the definitions at the end of the book is akin to unveiling the final pieces of a complex puzzle. It provides a sense of closure and clarity, allowing the reader to fully grasp the concepts and terminology introduced throughout the book. Use them to start a conversation with a friend about your own personal journey and the impact these factors have had on your life or as a springboard for your own continued research.

Anxiety is a feeling of unease caused by fear of danger or misfortune, often accompanied by physical symptoms such as rapid heartbeat or sweating. The opposite of anxiety isn't calm; it's safety. Feeling safe and secure is the antidote to anxiety. When individuals feel safe, they are able to relax and experience a sense of peace, allowing them to navigate life's challenges with greater ease. Creating a safe environment and cultivating a strong support system can help individuals combat anxiety and promote their overall mental well-being.

Anxious-Resistant is a type of attachment bond characterized by a constant need for reassurance and validation from their partner. These individuals often worry about being abandoned or rejected, leading them to become clingy or possessive in relationships. They may struggle with trust and have difficulty maintaining a sense of security, which can cause tension and conflict in their interactions with others.

Attachment Bond is the emotional connection and relationship between an infant and their primary caregiver. It is a critical aspect of early development and lays the foundation for future social and emotional interactions. This bond is characterized by trust, security, and comfort, providing the child a secure base to explore the world around them.

Authenticity allows us to fully embrace our flaws and imperfections and to let go of the need for external validation. It is the state of being true to oneself and expressing one's genuine thoughts, feelings, and beliefs. Embracing authenticity can lead to a sense of fulfillment and inner peace, as it encourages individuals to live in alignment with their values and true identity. It enables us to create a space for genuine connections and relationships where we can be accepted and loved for who we truly are. This not only improves well-being but also contributes to a more authentic and compassionate world where individuals feel safe to be themselves.

Autonomic Nervous System is an arm of the peripheral nervous system. It regulates involuntary bodily functions such as heart rate, digestion, and breathing. It is divided into two branches: the sympathetic nervous system, which prepares the body for "fight or flight" responses in stressful situations, and the parasympathetic nervous system, which promotes relaxation and restoration. The autonomic nervous system works in conjunction with the somatic nervous system to maintain homeostasis and ensure our body functions properly without conscious effort.

Avoidant Attachment is a type of attachment bond characterized by a fear of intimacy and a desire for independence. Individuals with an avoidant attachment style tend to prioritize their own needs and may struggle with emotional vulnerability. They may distance themselves from others to avoid potential rejection or hurt, making it challenging for them to form deep and meaningful connections. This attachment style can lead to a cycle of pushing others away and feeling lonely or isolated as a result.

Baader-Meinhof Phenomenon is a cognitive bias that occurs when a person learns or becomes aware of something and starts noticing it everywhere. It is also known as a frequency illusion. This phenomenon can make individuals feel like the occurrence of newly learned information has significantly increased when it is their perception that has changed.

Body Scan Meditation is a practice that can cultivate mindfulness and promote self-awareness. It involves systematically bringing attention to different parts of the body and noticing any sensations or tensions that may be present. This practice can help individuals develop a greater sense of connection with their bodies and become more attuned to their physical and emotional needs. Regularly engaging in body scan meditations can enhance overall well-being and promote personal growth.

BQ or Body Intelligence is the ability to understand and connect with one's body and interpret and respond to the physical signals it sends. It involves being in tune with bodily sensations and making choices that prioritize physical well-being. BQ also encompasses the capacity to listen to and respect the body's limits and engage in activities that promote health and vitality. Developing BQ can lead to improved self-care, increased energy levels, and greater overall well-being.

Burnout is a state of physical, emotional, or mental exhaustion caused by prolonged and excessive stress. It is characterized by feelings of cynicism, detachment, and a lack of motivation towards work or other activities. Burnout can also manifest in physical symptoms such as headaches, insomnia, and a weakened immune system. It is important to recognize the signs of burnout early and take steps to address it in order to prevent further negative consequences to one's well-being and overall quality of life.

Chronic Illness is a health condition or disease that is persistent or otherwise long-lasting. The term *chronic* is often applied when the course of the disease lasts for more than three months. A chronic condition usually affects multiple areas of the body, is not fully responsive to treatment, and persists for an extended period.

Compartmentalization is a defense mechanism in which thoughts and feelings that seem to conflict are kept separated or isolated from each other in the mind.

Compassion is the ability to understand and empathize with others, showing kindness and support. Practicing compassion has been found to have a positive impact on mental and physical health, as it can help reduce stress levels and promote feelings of happiness and well-being. By cultivating compassion, individuals can not only improve their own well-being but also contribute to creating a more compassionate and harmonious society.

Co-regulation involves the process of attuning to and responding to the emotions and needs of others in order to create a sense of safety, understanding, and connection. Co-regulation can be seen in various relationships, such as parent-child interactions, friendships, romantic partnerships, and professional counseling. By engaging in co-regulation, individuals can support each other's emotional well-being and foster healthier and more meaningful connections.

Conscious Awareness is the state of being fully present and engaged in the present moment without judgment or attachment to past or future events. It is the capacity to be aware of and comprehend your thoughts, feelings, and experiences without becoming overwhelmed by them. Developing a higher level of consciousness allows for greater self-awareness and the ability to make conscious choices that align with your values and goals.

Dashboard lights are to a car what symptoms are to the body. They serve as warning signs that something may be out of balance and require attention. Just like ignoring dashboard lights can lead to further damage to a car, ignoring or masking these flashing lights can potentially worsen health conditions or hinder personal growth.

***Dis*-ease** refers to any condition or state where the body's natural balance is disrupted, leading to physical or mental discomfort. Dis-ease can manifest in various forms, ranging from minor ailments to chronic illnesses, and can be caused by a multitude of factors such as genetics, lifestyle choices, or environmental influences.

Disorganized - Disoriented Attachment is a type of attachment bond characterized by a combination of both anxious and avoidant behaviors. Individuals with a disorganized attachment style may exhibit contradictory and unpredictable responses in relationships. They may have difficulty regulating their emotions and struggle with forming consistent patterns of attachment. This can lead to confusion and uncertainty in their relationships, as well as difficulties in trusting others or themselves.

EQ or Intellectual Intelligence is the ability to think critically, solve problems, and reason logically. It involves skills such as analyzing information, making sound judgments, and adapting to new situations. EQ also encompasses the capacity to understand and manage one's emotions and empathize with others. It plays a crucial role in effective communication, building relationships, and navigating social interactions. Developing EQ can lead to greater self-awareness, better decision-making, and improved overall well-being.

Excitotoxin is a substance that overstimulates nerve cells, leading to damage or death. Excitotoxins are often found in food additives, such as monosodium glutamate (MSG) and aspartame, and have been linked to various neurological disorders. These substances can trigger an excessive release of certain neurotransmitters, causing a cascade of events that can harm brain cells. It is important to be aware of the potential risks associated with excitotoxins and make informed choices about the foods we consume.

Fixed Mindset is a perspective characterized by the belief that abilities and intelligence are fixed traits that cannot be changed or developed. This mindset can lead to a lack of effort, avoidance of challenges, and a fear of failure. It hinders individuals from taking risks and embracing opportunities for growth and learning.

Glimmer is a micro-moment that fills us with optimism, a sense of safety, and belonging. Glimmers occur intermittently throughout the day; we simply have to look to find them. Social worker Deb Dana first used the word "glimmer" in her book The Polyvagal Theory in Therapy: Engaging the Rhythm of Regulation. It is thought to be the opposite of a trigger.

Gratitude is the deep appreciation and recognition of the positive aspects of life. It involves acknowledging the kindness and generosity of others, as well as expressing thankfulness for the blessings and opportunities that come our way. Gratitude is a powerful emotion that allows us to shift our perspective from dwelling on the negative to focusing on the good. It fosters a sense of contentment and happiness, enhancing our overall well-being and strengthening our relationships with others. Practicing gratitude can bring about a profound sense of fulfillment and create a ripple effect of positivity in both our personal lives and the world at large.

Growth Mindset is a perspective based on the belief that abilities and intelligence can be developed through dedication, effort, and learning. It is characterized by a willingness to take on challenges, a belief in the power of action, and resilience in the face of setbacks. A growth mindset allows individuals to embrace opportunities for personal growth and success, as they see failures as learning experiences rather than defining moments.

Health Continuum is a model also referred to as an *illness-wellness continuum*, is a visual tool that can be used to help people make healthy choices in their lives. At one end of the continuum is premature death, while optimal health lies at the other end.

Holistic Medicine is a form of healthcare that considers the physical, mental, emotional, and spiritual well-being of an individual. It emphasizes the importance of treating the person as a whole and not just focusing on specific symptoms or diseases. Holistic medicine often incorporates various alternative therapies and practices, such as acupuncture, herbal medicine, and mindfulness techniques, to promote overall health and wellness.

Inner-child is a concept referring to the unhealed and vulnerable aspects of our psyche that were formed during childhood experiences. It represents our authentic self, filled with innocence, curiosity, and creativity. Understanding and nurturing our inner child can lead to healing past wounds, increasing self-compassion, and fostering personal growth.

Limiting Belief is a belief that holds an individual back from reaching their full potential or achieving their goals. It is often rooted in fear, self-doubt, or negative past experiences. Limiting beliefs can create a fixed mindset and prevent personal growth and success.

Love is a force that can heal wounds, provide comfort during difficult times, and give meaning to life. When love is present, it has the power to transform individuals and the world around them, making it an essential aspect of human existence.

Macronutrients are nutrients the body needs in large quantities to provide calories or energy for daily functioning; otherwise known as Carbohydrates, Fats, and Proteins.

Micronutrients are also known as vitamins and minerals; they are needed in small quantities but are vital to healthy development, disease prevention, and well-being. Vitamins are necessary for energy production, immune function, blood clotting, and other functions. Minerals, known as our spark plugs, play an important role in growth, bone health, fluid balance, and several other processes.

Manifestation means turning your dreams, goals, and aspirations into reality by believing that you can achieve them while taking action steps toward that goal. The crucial aspect of this process is to align a belief with thoughts and energy in the form of action. In other words, setting clear intentions, visualizing success, and taking consistent action toward your goals. You cannot manifest something if there is something subconsciously holding you back.

Metta Meditation is a practice of cultivating loving-kindness and compassion towards oneself and others. It involves repeating specific phrases or mantras to generate feelings of goodwill and empathy. By directing positive intentions towards ourselves and all beings, Metta Meditation aims to promote inner peace, reduce negative emotions, and foster a sense of interconnectedness with the world around us. This practice can be done individually or in a group setting, and it is believed to have numerous benefits for mental well-being and overall happiness.

Mind-body Connection is the idea that there is a strong link between the thoughts and emotions of the mind and the physical health and well-being of the body. This connection suggests that our mental state can influence our physical health and vice versa. By recognizing and nurturing this connection, individuals can improve their overall well-being by practicing mindfulness, engaging in stress-reducing activities, and adopting healthy habits such as exercise and proper nutrition.

Mirror Neurons are specialized cells in the brain that fire both when an individual performs an action and when they observe someone else performing the same action. This phenomenon allows individuals to understand and empathize with others, as well as learn new skills through observation. Mirror neurons have been linked to various social behaviors, such as imitation, empathy, and understanding others' intentions.

Multidimensional means having different facets, elements, or factors.

Naturopathic Doctors combine traditional medical knowledge with natural therapies and approaches to promote healing and overall wellness. They focus on treating the root cause of illnesses rather than just managing symptoms, using a holistic approach that takes into account the physical, mental, and emotional aspects of a person's health. Naturopathic Doctors may use various treatments such as herbal medicine, nutrition counseling, acupuncture, and lifestyle modifications to support the body's natural healing abilities.

Nervous System is a bodily system that allows us to experience and respond to life's stimuli. It is a complex network of nerves and cells that transmit signals between different parts of the body. This system is responsible for coordinating and controlling all bodily functions, including movement, sensation, and cognition. Additionally, the nervous system is divided into two main parts: the central nervous system (CNS) and the peripheral nervous system (PNS). The CNS consists of the brain and spinal cord, while the PNS includes all the nerves that connect the CNS to other parts of the body.

Nervous System Dysregulation occurs when your nervous system enters an indefinite state of survival, signaling danger throughout your body when there is no life-threatening danger.

Primary Control is an individual's ability to influence and shape their environment to meet their needs and desires. It involves taking charge of one's own actions and actively seeking out opportunities for personal growth and fulfillment.

Resiliency is the ability to bounce back from adversity and adapt to challenges. It involves developing a strong mindset and coping skills to effectively navigate difficult situations. Building resiliency can help individuals better manage stress, maintain a positive outlook, and recover from setbacks more quickly.

Resistance is the unconscious defense mechanism that individuals use to protect themselves from uncomfortable or threatening thoughts, emotions, or experiences. It often manifests as a reluctance or refusal to engage with certain ideas or behaviors that may challenge one's existing beliefs or ways of thinking.

Resonance is a vibrational frequency emitted by our cells, organs, and systems. By tuning ourselves into the energetic frequencies of our own being, we can tap into the innate wisdom of our bodies and cultivate a greater sense of self-awareness and connection with the world around us.

Secondary Control is the ability to adapt and find meaning in situations that are beyond an individual's control. It involves accepting and making the best of circumstances rather than trying to change them. Secondary control allows individuals to maintain a sense of inner peace and contentment, even when faced with challenges or setbacks.

Secure Attachment is a type of attachment bond characterized by a healthy and balanced approach to relationships. Individuals with a secure attachment style are typically able to trust others, form deep emotional connections, and feel secure in their relationships. They are less likely to push people away or sabotage their relationships, as they have a strong sense of self-worth and believe in the stability of their connections.

Self-regulation refers to the ability to manage and control one's thoughts, emotions, and behaviors to promote overall well-being. Self-regulation techniques such as deep breathing exercises, meditation, and positive self-talk can help individuals maintain a healthy mental and physical health balance. By practicing self-regulation, individuals can reduce stress levels, improve their mood, and enhance their overall quality of life.

Silos in Business can be described as a lack of communication and collaboration between different departments or groups. Silos can hinder productivity, innovation, and overall organizational success. They can create a sense of isolation and prevent the sharing of knowledge and resources. Breaking down silos requires a concerted effort to foster open communication, encourage cross-functional collaboration, and promote a culture of teamwork and inclusivity. By doing so, organizations can harness the collective talents and expertise of their employees, leading to improved efficiency, creativity, and overall success.

Silos in Healthcare can be described as the divisions and barriers that exist between different departments or specialties within a healthcare organization. These silos can hinder effective communication and collaboration, leading to fragmented patient care and missed opportunities for innovation and improvement. Breaking down silos in healthcare requires a shift towards a more integrated and collaborative approach, where healthcare professionals from different disciplines work together towards common goals, share information and resources, and prioritize the needs of patients above departmental boundaries. This can result in improved patient outcomes, increased efficiency, and a more holistic approach.

Spirit is a person's inner essence. It encompasses their beliefs, values, and attitudes and is often associated with qualities such as resilience, determination, and optimism. Spirituality can also refer to a connection with something greater than oneself, whether it be a higher power, nature, or the universe. It can provide individuals with a sense of purpose and meaning in life, guiding their actions and decisions. Nurturing one's spirit can lead to personal fulfillment and a deeper understanding of oneself and the world.

Somatic Nervous System is an arm of the peripheral nervous system responsible for controlling voluntary movements and transmitting sensory information to the CNS. It consists of sensory neurons that carry information from the body's senses to the CNS, as well as motor neurons that transmit signals from the CNS to muscles, allowing for voluntary movement. The somatic nervous system plays a crucial role in our ability to interact with and navigate our environment. It also works in conjunction with the autonomic nervous system to maintain homeostasis and ensure our body functions properly without conscious effort.

Subconscious is the part of the mind that operates below the level of conscious awareness, influencing thoughts, feelings, and behaviors. It is responsible for automatic processes such as habits, instincts, and intuition. Understanding the subconscious can provide insight into underlying motivations and help individuals make positive changes in their lives.

Symptoms are signs or messages from the body that let us know something is out of alignment. They can manifest in various ways, such as physical discomfort, emotional distress, or behavioral changes. Understanding symptoms is crucial in identifying and addressing underlying issues, whether they are related to health, mental well-being, or personal relationships. By recognizing and interpreting symptoms, individuals can take proactive steps toward seeking appropriate help and finding solutions to improve their overall quality of life.

Trauma is an emotional response to a distressing event or experience that overwhelms an individual's ability to cope. Trauma can vary significantly from person to person, resulting from a wide range of experiences. Trauma can have long-lasting effects on a person's mental and physical health, often leading to symptoms such as anxiety, depression, and difficulty forming and maintaining relationships. It is important for individuals who have experienced trauma to seek support in order to heal and regain a sense of safety and well-being.

Quantum Biofeedback is a non-invasive therapeutic technology that energetically scans and harmonizes the body's stresses and imbalances. A scientifically proven method for reducing stress in the body. Stressors include allergens, bacteria, viruses, emotional stress, and pain.

Ultra-Processed Food is a category of food that goes through extensive processing and contains additives, preservatives, and artificial ingredients. These foods are often high in calories, unhealthy fats, sugar, and sodium. They are typically low in essential nutrients like fiber, vitamins, and minerals. Regular consumption of ultra-processed foods has been linked to an increased risk of obesity, heart disease, and other chronic health conditions.

Vagus Nerve is known as the wandering nerve because it has multiple branches that extend from the brainstem to various organs in the body, including the heart, lungs, and digestive system. It is a crucial part of the parasympathetic nervous system, which is responsible for controlling rest and digest functions. The vagus nerve plays a crucial role in regulating many bodily functions, such as heart rate, digestion, and even mood. Additionally, the vagus nerve is involved in the body's response to stress and helps to promote relaxation and calmness. When it is out of balance, it can lead to various health issues, such as gastrointestinal disorders, heart problems, and mood disorders. Dysregulation of the vagus nerve can also contribute to symptoms like anxiety, depression, and chronic fatigue.

Therefore, maintaining healthy vagus nerve function is essential for overall well-being and optimal bodily functions.

Wellness Ecology is a way of thinking that considers the interconnected impact of internal and external variables on health and well-being. Each and every facet of our existence has an impact on us, positively or negatively. By taking this approach, one can appreciate the many aspects that influence health and happiness. By adopting this tack, we gain the agency to make thoughtful decisions to foster a more positive and healthful environment.

Chapter 15

Notes for Reference

It's an Inside Job was crafted over 18 months and a lifetime; what follows does not strive to be an exhaustive chronicle of every influence on our thoughts. Instead, it stands as a catalog of what we deem the most pivotal sources for this book. Recognizing our humanity, we welcome your outreach for corrections if omissions or inaccuracies are apparent. Please feel free to contact us at: info@sevendimensions.org

CHAPTER TWO - THE SEVEN DIMENSIONS

This framework was originally conceptualized in 1979 by Dr. Aaron Antonovsky: Fig. 11.3, [The ease/dis-ease continuum (Antonovsky,). . .]. - The Handbook of Salutogenesis, NCBI Bookshelf. (n.d.). Fig. 11.3, [the Ease/Dis-ease Continuum (Anton-Ovsky), ovsky,)the Handbook of Salutogenesis - NCBI Bookshelf. gov/books/NBK435812/figure/ch11.Fig3/

The World Health Organization (WHO) stated, as early as 1948: Constitution of the World Health Organization. In: World Health Organization: Basic documents. 45th ed. Geneva: World Health Organization; 2005.

In 1976, Dr. Bill Hettler, co-founder of the National Wellness Institute (NWI), identified Six Dimensions of Wellness: Six Dimensions of Wellness—National Wellness Institute. (2020, April 29). National

Wellness Institute. https://nationalwellness.org/resources/six-dimensions-of-wellness/

Instead, we identify with Dr. Lissa Rankin's health cairn, where the physical dimension sits on top: The Whole Health Cairn: A Radical New Wellness Model. (n.d.). Lissa Rankin. https:// lissarankin.com/the-whole-health-cairn-a-radical-new-wellness-model/

"To be "well" is not to live in a state of perpetual safety and calm but to move fluidly from a state of adversity, risk, adventure, or excitement back to safety and calm and out again." —Emily Nagoski: Nagoski, E., & Nagoski, A. (2020, January 7). Burn-out: The Secret to Unlocking the Stress Cycle. Ballantine Books.

"Make new friends but keep the old; one is silver and the other's gold.": Fleming, V (Director). (1939). *The Wizard of Oz.* Metro-Goldwyn-Mayer

According to Dr. Kelly McGonigal, health psychologist and lecturer at Stanford University, stress can build resiliency, boost cognitive function, and act as a powerful motivator if we learn to use it to our advantage: University, S. (2015, May 7). Embracing stress is more important than reducing stress, Stanford psychologist says. Stanford News. https://news.stanford.edu/2015/05/07/ stress-embrace-mcgonigal-050715/

As described in an article for Well+Good, Neuroscientist and mental health specialist Caroline Leaf, Ph.D., says that after an event, there will be an initial biochemical and electrical spike lasting 30 to 90 seconds where our unconscious and conscious mind adapts and digests the incoming information: Estrada, J. (2022, April 7). 5 Ways To Regulate Your Nervous System, According to a Neuroscientist | Well+Good. Well+Good. regulate-your-nervous-system/

CHAPTER THREE - INTELLECTUAL

Let's begin our discussion of this dimension with some fun facts about the brain. This complex organ comprises about 2% of the body's total weight but uses 20% of its energy and oxygen intake. Weighing about three pounds, it's the fattiest organ in the body: S. (2019, February 23). 72 Amazing Human Brain Facts (Based on the Latest Science) San Diego Brain Injury Foundation. San Diego Brain Injury Foundation. https://sdbif. org/72-amazing-human-brain-facts-based-on-the-latest-science/

The brain is 73% water, and even the slightest bit of dehydration affects attention, memory, and other cognitive skill: Our 3 brains—Why 95% of Our Behaviors Are Not Conscious (Extended Review). (2021, December 13). Lifestyle Medicine With Rory Callaghan. https://www.rorycal- laghan.com/our-3-brains-why-95-of-our-behaviors-are-not-conscious/

According to Dr. Joe Dispenza, neuroscientist, researcher, and chiropractor, "95% of who we are by the time we're 35 years old is a memorized set of behaviors, emotional reactions, unconscious habits, hardwired attitudes, beliefs, and perceptions that function like a computer program.": The Official Website of Dr Joe Dispenza. (n.d.). Unlimited With Dr Joe Dispenza. https://drjoedispenza.com/

Eckhart Tolle believes we should not identify with our thoughts but rather observe them: https://eckhart-tolle-essential-teachings.simplecast.com/episodes/watch-your-mind

"When you make a choice, you change the future." Chopra, D. (1994, November 9). The Seven Spiritual Laws of Success: A Practical Guide to the Fulfillment of Your Dreams.

This type of experience is called the Baader- Meinhof phenomenon, also known as the frequency illusion or frequency bias:

Nikolopoulou, K. (2022, November 2). The Baader–Meinhof Phenomenon Explained. Scribbr. .com/r

The mind gives rise to 48.6 thoughts per minute, or 70,000 daily, according to the Laboratory of Neuro Imaging at the University of Southern California: Laboratory of NeuroImaging. (2023, February 21). Laboratory of NeuroImaging. https://loni.usc.edu/

A growth mindset is one of this dimension's most important indicators for optimal health. Carol Dweck, a Stanford University psychologist, found people are influenced by two perspectives—growth and fixed: University, S. (2021, September 16). Your powerful, changeable mindset—Stanford Report. Stanford Report.

A woman's risk of getting this deadly disease during her lifetime is about 1 in 78: Fast Facts from the WHA Information Center: September is Gynecologic Cancer Awareness Month. (n.d.). WHA - Fast Facts From the WHA Information Center: September Is Gynecologic Cancer Awareness Month.

Gabor Maté, MD, author of *When the Body Says No,* says that we could prevent and heal many diseases if we fully understood the scientific evidence that shows the mind and body are one: Maté, G., & Maté, G. (2011, January 1). *When the Body Says No: Exploring the Stress-Disease Connection.*

CHAPTER FOUR - EMOTIONAL

According to Dr. Jill Bolte Taylor, a Harvard-trained and published neuroscientist, 90 seconds is all it takes for an emotion to move through the body and dissipate. "When a person has a reaction to something in their environment, there's a 90-second chemical process that happens in the body; any remaining emotional response is just the person choosing to stay in that emotional loop,"

she explains: Taylor, J. B. (2009, May 26). *My Stroke of Insight: A Brain Scientist's Personal Journey.* Penguin Books.

The term Emotional Intelligence first appeared in the early 1960s but gained popularity with the book by psychologist Daniel Goleman, Ph.D., *Emotional Intelligence: Why It Can Matter More Than IQ.:* Emotional intelligence (emotional quotient or EQ) can help us connect with our feelings and build stronger relationships: Goleman, D. (2005, September 27). *Emotional Intelligence: Why It Can Matter More Than IQ.* Bantam.

According to Dr. Peter Levine, in his book Waking the Tiger, animals use shaking to release trauma energy from their bodies. The stress cycle has a beginning, middle, and end: Ergos Institute, inc TM. (n.d.). Ergos Institute, IncTM. https://www.somaticexperiencing.com

CHAPTER FIVE - SOCIAL

According to Dr. Leaf, Ph.D., as we co-regulate with someone, mirror neurons in the brain are activated, enabling the person in the deregulated state to literally "mirror" calmness: How Co-Regulation Can Help Build Self-Regulation Skills. (n.d.). Dr. Leaf. https://drleaf.com/blogs/news/how-co-regulation-can-help-build-self-regulation-skills

"Being able to feel safe with other people is probably the single most important aspect of mental health; safe connections are fundamental to meaningful and satisfying lives.": der Kolk, B. V. (2014, September 25). The Body Keeps the Score: Brain, Mind, and Body in the Healing of Trauma. Viking.

According to British psychiatrist John Bowlby and American psychologist Mary Ainsworth, the bonding quality we experience

during this first relationship often determines how well we relate to other people and respond to intimacy throughout life: The Origins of Attachment Theory. John Bowlby and Mary Ainsworth, Inge Brether- ton, Developmental Psychology (1992), 28, 759-775 e du/attachment/online/inge_origins.pdf

According to holistic psychologist Dr. Nicole LePera, learning which early attachment style resonates most with you can help make these connections: LePera, N. (2021, March 9). How to Do the Work: Recognize Your Patterns, Heal from Your Past, and Create Your Self. Harper Wave.

Many trace the concept of our inner child to psychiatrist Carl Jung, who described a child archetype in his work: Child Archetype - Wikipedia. (2012, May 21). Child Archetype - Wikipedia. https://en .wikipedia.org/wiki/Child_archetype

According to the Mayo Clinic, social anxiety is more than everyday nervousness; it includes fear, anxiety, and avoidance that interferes with relationships, daily routines, work, school, or other activities: .Socialanxietydisorder(socialphobia)—Symptomsandcauses.(2021,June19).MayoClinic. causes/syc-20353561

Russell Kennedy, MD, a neuroscientist and the author of *Anxiety Rx,* claims that all anxiety is separation anxiety or an intense fear of being cut off from one's SELF: Kennedy, R. (2020, October 15). Anxiety Rx: A New Prescription for Anxiety Relief from the Doctor Who Created It.

"Make new friends but keep the old; one is silver and the other's gold." - Parry, J. (N.D.) 'New Friends and Old Friends'

CHAPTER SIX - ENVIRONMENTAL

We are big fans of Daphne Miller, MD, author of *Farmacology, Total Health from the Ground Up.* Dr. Miller left her medical practice on a nationwide research project to examine what farming can teach us about nurturing and healing ourselves; how cool is that? She explains that the key to successful production is to give more attention to the farm than any particular product it may yield: Miller, D. (2013, April 16). *Farmacology: Total Health from the Ground Up.* William Morrow & Company.

According to the Centers for Disease Control (CDC), chronic disease is the leading cause of death and disability in the U.S. and costs the nation $4.1 trillion in annual healthcare costs. Six in 10 adults have a chronic disease, and four in 10 have two or more: .About Chronic Diseases | CDC. (2022, July 21). About Chronic Diseases | CDC.

Life Expectancy in the U.S. Dropped for the Second Year in a Row in 2021. (2022, August 31). Life Expectancy in the U.S. Dropped for the Second Year in a Row in 2021.

FAS are found in many household products, the CDC estimates that 97% of Americans have some level of PFAS in their blood: PFAS in the US population | ATSDR. (2022, December 22). PFAS in the US Population | ATSDR.

Rather than homemade bread, we used a popular store-bought version that contained calcium propionate (C.P.). C.P. is one of the many additives used in processed baked goods to extend shelf life: Robinson, J., Flores, R., Johansson, R., Bloomfield, F., & Sky, Z. (2019, February 15). Calcium Propionate—toxicity, side effects, diseases, and environmental impacts. Natural Pedia Com. facts-diseases-and-envir onmental-impacts.html

American women use 12 personal care products that contain 168 different chemicals: The Toxic Twelve Chemicals and Contaminants in Cosmetics. (n.d.). Environmental Working Group. https://www.ewg.org/sites/default/files/u352/Toxic%2020%20List.pdf

According to the National Library of Medicine, although the skin may have served as the entry point, endocrine disruption results from exposure. Several ingredients in sunscreens, cosmetics, and personal care products have endocrine-active properties that can affect reproductive health and lead to cancer: Cosmetics as endocrine disruptors: are they a health risk? —PubMed. (2015, December 1). PubMed.

Environmental Working Group (EWG). Best known for their annual Clean 15 and Dirty Dozen, EWG's mission is to empower us with breakthrough research to make informed choices and live healthier lives in a healthier environment: EWG. Group, E. W. (2023, March 21). EWG's 2023 Shopper's Guide to Pesticides in ProduceTM. EWG's 2023 Shopper's Guide to Pesticides in Produce.

Valisure. (2021, May 25). Valisure. e-news-sure-detects-benzene-in-sunscreen

Aluminum's possible connection to breast cancer, breast cysts, and Alzheimer's disease has raised some concerns in the medical community: Darbre P, Mannello F, Exley C. Aluminium and breast cancer: Sources of exposure, tissue measurements and mechanisms of toxicological actions on breast biology. J Inorg Biochem. 2013; 128: 257-261

In the February 2023 newsletter published by Hidden Brain..., Shankar Vedantam asks, "Would we spend less time on social media if it were more sociable?": Vedantam, S. (n.d.). A Small but Effective Way to Fight Loneliness. https://news.hiddenbrain.org/p/a-small-but-effective-way-to-fight

In discussing taking control of our thoughts, three notable examples came to mind: Louie Zamperini, prisoner of war: Louis Zamperini:

From Olympic Track Star to POW. VA News. (2019, November 14). VA News. https://news.va.gov/68125/louis-zamperini-from-olympic-track-star-to-pow/

Victor Frankl, holocaust survivor and author of *Man's Search for Meaning:* Frankl, V. E. (2006, June 1). Man's Search for Meaning. Beacon Press.

Nelson Mandela, who went from prisoner to the first black president of South Africa.: Nelson Mandela—Wikipedia. (2013, December 17). Nelson Mandela - Wikipedia. https://en.wikipedia.org/wiki/Nelson_Mandela

"When your environment is clean, you feel happy, motivated, and healthy." Lailah Gifty .com. .com/ Dr. Mark Hyman. (n.d.). Dr. Mark Hyman. https://drhyman.com/

CHAPTER SEVEN - OCCUPATIONAL

In the working paper *Children and Gender Inequality: Evidence From Denmark,* by Henrik Kleven, Camille Landais, and Jakob Egholt Søgaard, the authors explore how women are influenced by the examples set by their mothers: Kleven, H., Landais, C., & Søgaard, J. E. (n.d.). Children and Gender Inequality: Evidence from Denmark. American Economic Association. Children and Gender Inequality: Evidence From Denmark. American Economic Association.

But how is a child's mental health affected by their parent's careers? To answer that question, we turned to a study by Stewart D. Friedman, an organizational psychologist at the Wharton School, and Jeff Greenhaus from Drexel University: How Our Careers Affect Our Children. (2018, November 14). Harvard Business Review. https://hbr.org/2018/11/how-our-careers-affect-our-children

According to Dr. Ricky Fernandez, PT, DPT, Burnout Coach, the number one sign of burnout is emotional exhaustion: Instagram. https://www.instagram.com/ricky_theburnoutcoach/

According to a 2021 study conducted by Oracle and Workplace Intelligence, an HR research and advisory firm, 75% of respondents feel professionally trapped, and 29% said they are struggling financially. But, maybe most alarming is that 28% indicated they suffer from worsening mental health, and 23% feel detached from their own lives: 82% of People Believe Robots Can Support Their Career Better Than Humans. (n.d.). Oracle.

January 2023 survey by LendingClub indicates 60% of U.S . consumers say they're living paycheck to paycheck: 60% of Americans Now Living Paycheck to Paycheck, Down from 64% a Month Ago. (2023, February 28). 60% of Americans Now Living Paycheck to Paycheck, Down From 64% a Month Ago | LendingClub Corporation. https://ir.lendingclub. com/news/news-details/2023/60-of-Americans-Now-Living-Paycheck-to-Paycheck- Down-from-64-a-Month-Ago/default.aspx

Deb encouraged Diane to read *Emotional Intelligence: Why It Can Matter More Than IQ,* by Daniel Goleman, Ph.D.: Goleman, D. (2005, September 27). *Emotional Intelligence: Why It Can Matter More Than IQ.* Bantam.

CHAPTER EIGHT - SPIRITUAL

She can feel her dad whenever she hears the Emerson, Lake & Palmer song "Lucky Man": Lake, Greg. "Lucky Man." Emerson Lake & Palmer. Cotillion Records, 1970. Record.

Jack Kornfield, spiritual teacher and author of *A Path with Heart*, shares, "The things that matter most in our lives are not fantastic or grand. They are the moments when we touch one another and when we are there in the most caring way. This simple and profound intimacy is the love that we all long for.": Kornfield, J. (2009, May 19). *The Wise Heart: A Guide to the Universal Teachings of Buddhist Psychology*. Bantam.

CHAPTER NINE - PHYSICAL

...**new outer layer of skin every month**: Epidermis and Its Renewal by Stem Cells-Molecular Biology of the Cell. NCBI Bookshelf. Epidermis and Its Renewal by Stem Cells. Molecular Biology of the Cell. https://www.ncbi.nlm.nih.gov/books/NBK26865/#:~:text=Skin%20consists%20of%20a%20tough,the%20order%20of%20a%20month.

...and a new skeleton every 10 years: Bone Health Basics-OrthoInfo-AAOS. (2020, May 1). Bone Health Basics-OrthoInfo-AAOS. https://www.orthoinfo.org/en/staying-healthy/bone-health-basics/

In addition, our stomach lining renews every four to five days to prevent the stomach from digesting itself. Understanding how the intestine replaces and repairs itself. (2017, July 14). Harvard Gazette. https://news.harvard.edu/gazette/story/2017/07/understanding-how-the-intestine-replaces-and-repairs-itself/

Did you know that the number of bacteria in the body may be similar to the number of human cells?: NIH Human Microbiome Project defines the normal bacterial makeup of the body. (2015, August 31). National Institutes of Health (NIH). Events/news-releases/nih-human-microbiome-project-defines-normal-bacterial-makeup-body

Two to six pounds of bacteria inhabit the digestive tract of a human, and they play a crucial role in digestion, immunity, and even mental health.: Introduction to the human gut microbiota https://www.ncbi.nlm.nih.gov/pmc/articles/PMC5433529/

Estimates suggest that 20% of the world's population suffers from chronic pain on a daily basis.: Goldberg, D. S., & McGee, S. J. (2011, October 6). Pain as a global public health priority. PubMed Central (PMC).

According to Dr. Bradley Nelson, author of *The Emotion Code:* these trapped emotions can build up, causing pain, dysfunction, and disease. Nelson, B. (2019, June 1). *The Emotion Code: How to Release Your Trapped Emotions for Abundant Health, Love, and Happiness* (Updated and Expanded Edition). St. Martin's Essentials.

According to Dr. Eli Jarrouge, most metabolic health benefits come from what you STOP eating: .Meet Dr. Elie Jarrouge | Metabolic Health MD. (n.d.). Metabolic Health MD. https://www.metabolichealthmd.com/eliejarrouge

What do you do between 12 and 20 times a minute and 17,000 to 30,000 times a day, and you probably don't even realize you're doing it?: https://www.nm.org/healthbeat/healthy-tips/4-breathing-techniques-for-better-health

Journalist James Nestor, the author of the eye-opening book *Breath,* travels the world to figure out what went wrong and how to fix it: .Nestor, J. (2020, May 26). *Breath: The New Science of a Lost Art.* Riverhead Books. Podcast Archive. (n.d.). Ask The Dentist. https://askthedentist.com/podcast/

...according to Dr. Mark Burhenne, from the podcast *Ask the Dentist* with Dr. Mark Burhenne, even cavities and crooked teeth: Ask the Dentist, Health Begins in your mouth, https://askthedentist.com/

Amy Scher, author of How to Heal Yourself When No One Else Can offers a few common metaphors to consider when symptoms arise in certain body parts: Scher, A. B. (2016, January 8). How to Heal Yourself When No One Else Can: A Total Self-Healing Approach for Mind, Body, and Spirit.

Emerging evidence is showing that the gut-brain axis is one of the most powerful relationships in our body. The gut-brain axis: interactions between enteric microbiota, central and enteric nervous systems: Journal List Ann Gastroenterol v.28(2); https://www.ncbi.nlm.nih.gov/pmc/articles/PMC4367209/#:~:text=Strong%20evidence%20suggests%20that%20gut,response%2C%20anxiety%20and%20memory%20function

Chapter 16

About the Authors

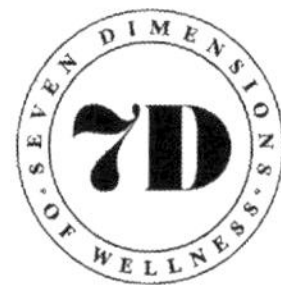

On a mission to spark curiosity toward a deeper understanding of what it means to be well.

The universe first united the authors to create a curriculum-based wellness book for the Healing Meals Community Project, a Connecticut-based nonprofit. Together, they wrote and designed *The NEW Book (Nutrition, Education, and Wellness: The Healing Meals Way),* a beautifully illustrated book that brings nourishment to life so that clients and volunteers can learn more about whole food nutrition and the relationship between diet, health outcomes, connection, and a sustainable environment.

While this trio followed very different paths in the wellness industry, they discovered that, despite their diverse backgrounds, their deepest desires were very much the same. They share a passion for promoting holistic well-being and recognize the importance of bringing authenticity and genuine care into their connections.

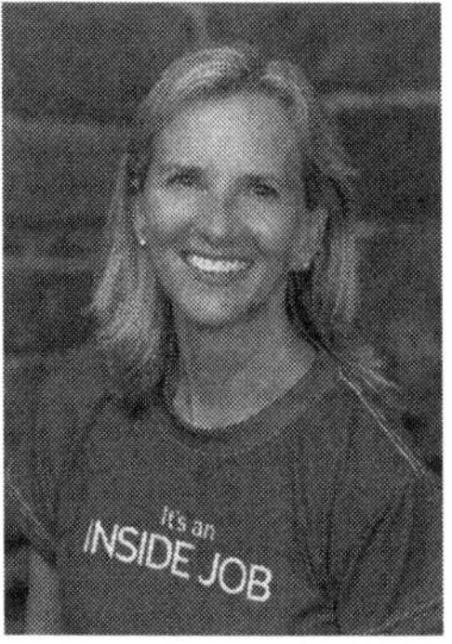

Tracy Arnold sees life as one big experiment. She embraces each day with an open mind and an appetite for growth and discovery. Her determination to overcome a chronic illness sparked an insatiable curiosity about what prevents and promotes the body's natural healing processes. Tracy is adept in holistic wellness, with a gift for empowering others to believe anything is possible. Arnold's approach is multidimensional, going beyond physical health to cover wellness concepts across all facets of life. She is a co-founder of Seven Dimensions of Wellness, an author, a certified yoga instructor, and an Institute for Integrative Nutrition-certified health and wellness coach. Tracy is a natural educator who encourages people to develop a closer connection with themselves and the world around them. Affectionately referred to as "Chief Fun Officer" by her partners, Tracy lives up to the title with her quick smile, easy laugh, and sincere desire to bring sunshine into everything she does.

Tracy@SevenDimensions.org

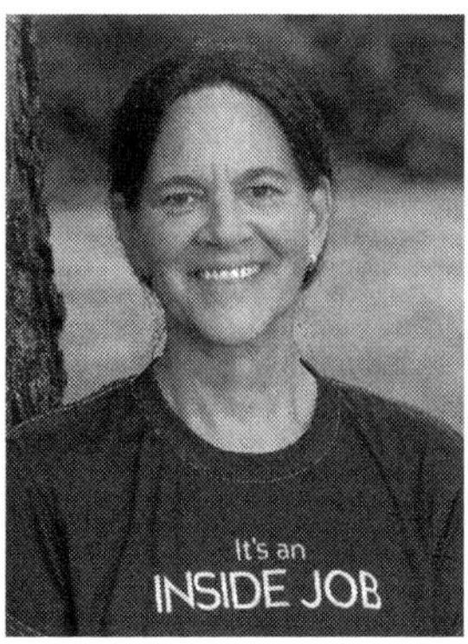

Helen Barnard's world changed dramatically when she began to see herself through a more compassionate lens. After using her creative talents for 25 years in NYC's magazine industry, Helen bought a farmhouse in Connecticut and returned to school to earn her master's degree in counseling. Using her own developmental experiences as inspiration to help others, she traded her artistic talents and impressive print skills to make the world a better place. Helen, a co-founder of Seven Dimensions of Wellness, is skilled in somatic experiencing and approaches therapy from a body-centered perspective. Her capacity for genuine connection enables others to embrace the whole of who they are. Her voice is soothing, and her shared experiences are honest, funny, and sometimes heartbreaking. You feel grateful for the chance to sit and listen as if you've stumbled upon a hidden treasure.

Helen@SevenDimensions.org

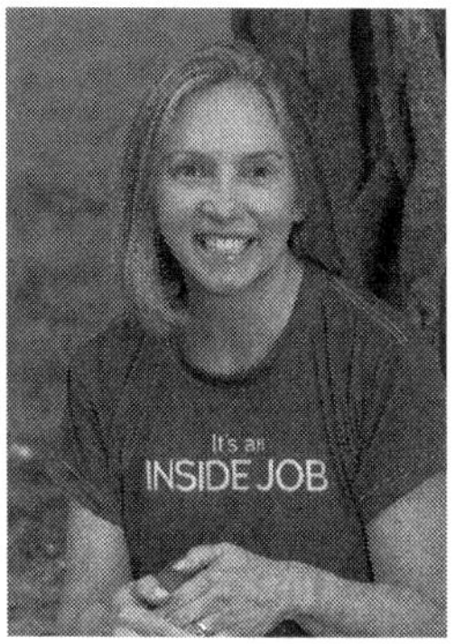

Diane Hubbard considers any challenge life throws her as an opportunity to dig deeper. She is an author, a co-founder of Seven Dimensions of Wellness, and a lifelong learner who is always looking to discover more. Diane worked in the financial services industry for 26 years, leading, learning, and growing. Her desire to make a difference in the world led her to work in the non-profit sector, where she spent over ten years demonstrating how to harness passion to deliver on missions effectively. She currently works as a consultant for organizations wanting to make a positive impact. Like Charlie Puth's song, "One Call Away," Superman has nothing on Diane. She is a defender and protector who inspires others to realize they are stronger than they think. The song highlights the importance of having someone to rely on during tough times, and Diane embodies that kind of support for those around her. Her unwavering strength and compassion make Diane inspiring to work with.

Diane@SevenDimensions.org

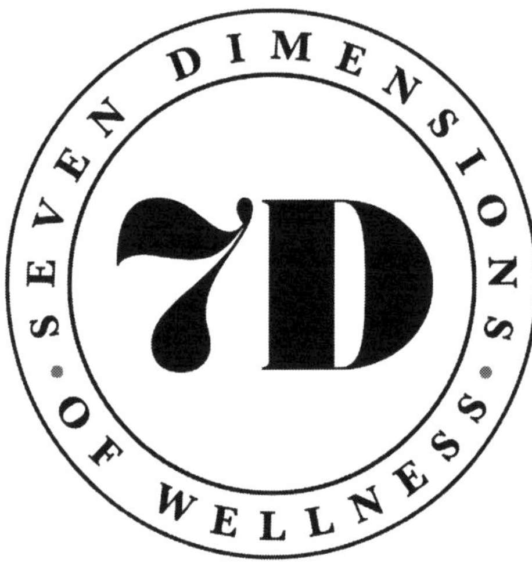

sevendimensions.org

Whatever you are
not changing,
you are choosing.

Made in the USA
Middletown, DE
29 May 2024